Hearing Loss
from stigma to strategy

Michael Simmons

PETER OWEN
LONDON AND CHESTER SPRINGS

PETER OWEN PUBLISHERS
73 Kenway Road, London SW5 0RE

First published in Great Britain 2005
by Peter Owen Publishers

A catalogue record for this book is available
from the British Library

ISBN 0 7206 1224 1

Printed and bound in Great Britain by
MPG Books Ltd, Bodmin, Cornwall

CONTENTS

By way of introduction

T O BE HONEST, this has been a highly complicated book to write. It started as one about suppressed anger and fear on a scale I had not contemplated before. It was to discuss the destruction of something I had always thought indestructible. I was thinking that I would linger on the losing of those threads of spontaneity, which as a healthy hearing person I had always taken for granted, and that I would reflect on the erosion and the spoiling of the intimacies with other people that hearing loss had brought about. And I was going to brood on the distortion of sound, all sound, that has now become part of my life, including the loss of quiet music and the clear singing of birds.

To some extent, that has been done. For certain, part of it has been implicitly about the emergence of an increasingly withdrawn, self-centred, impatient and grumpy old man – someone I didn't know before and a person who, I think, previously had a reputation for being hearty and good-humoured. He was someone who used to enjoy parties and social occasions, who loved theatre and concert-going and who was probably generally popular in his chosen peer groups. Friends and relatives, fellow journalists, fellow (mature) students, fellow lip-readers and cricketers seemed to accept this person and to like his company, just as he liked being with them.

But then, about halfway through the labour (or was it the therapy?) of writing the book, a door opened and it became a book about a search, which has been pretty successful, for lights at the end of the tunnel and, eventually, about recognizing some unexpected compensations for what has been lost. There is now, without a doubt, a new quality in the quiet moments that can still be had with close friends, in the uninterrupted conversations with my wife Angela and with my children and grand-children – even though it was the grandchildren who once dubbed me

Grumpy Grandad. Quiet moments were, of course, always accessible when you knew how and where to find them; now there seem to be more of them.

This remains unambiguously a book about hearing loss or what in audiological circles is known as acquired or age-related hearing loss, a condition which some family doctors have been known to dismiss as being – precisely because it is age related – untreatable. It is about deafness in the *Oxford Dictionary* sense that deafness is about being 'wholly or partly unable to hear', but the emphasis here is not so much on those who are wholly impaired as on those who are partly so. The line has to be drawn somewhere, but, inevitably, there are overlaps. In several contexts, and despite semantic protestations from the purists, it is convenient that people who are deaf and people who have hearing loss should be treated together. Their individual conditions and their needs may be very different, but there are many organizations offering treatment, therapy and support of all sorts, who have them in the same in-tray. Besides, the hearing world, unthinkingly, tends to think of them as being in the same sort of category.

This book is a wake-up nudge, rather than a wake-up call, as well as a gesture of support for those who used, more frequently, to be labelled hard of hearing. I am not a member of a hard-of-hearing club – perhaps I should be – and I don't go on organized coach trips to the seaside – and perhaps I should – partly because these clubs are fewer in number than they used to be and the ones near where I live don't do things I'm really interested in. Television, with enhanced sound and subtitles, seems to have taken over. However, I do quietly rejoice in the fact I have found and joined a new community, however ill-defined, which I knew almost nothing about before. I have, for a start, become a member of a local lip-reading group. To the uninitiated that may sound rather twee; but to the initiated there can be no doubt that it has become a very important and delightfully therapeutic fact of life.

Nothing too unusual in any of this. Millions of people have hearing loss, and a large proportion of them have come to endure it with endless reserves of stoicism they probably didn't know they had. What they may think about their condition when they are alone with their thoughts is not easy to determine, although I have been able to gain some insights in that highly sensitive area with my researches. But for many of them this particular loss may be just another unwelcome but inevitable symptom of the ageing process, something that has to be accepted with as good grace as one can muster. It comes along with the fallible memory, the wrinkles and the grey-then-white hairs that come to almost all of us – if they don't fall out first. These are things that simply happen when we get over the hill of something called middle age.

There are many disabilities and infirmities that, I have been told (several times), are worse than hearing loss. That may well be true, although it is as philosophically difficult as it is notionally unhelpful to compare one impairment, disability or handicap with another. Each of them brings its own share of sometimes very distinct disadvantages. Anyway, disability, to whatever degree, is what you make of it.

It is a familiar truth to anyone who has pondered for more than a moment on the subject of physical deterioration that, while the loss of sight cuts you off from seeing things and from savouring subtle variations of tone, colour and light and shade, the loss of hearing is something which cuts you off from people. You learn something new not only about loneliness but also about the inaccessibility of familiar things that have now been placed, sometimes quite unpredictably, beyond reach. The fact of being cut off was underlined during her hyperactive life by the American writer, academic and social reformer Helen Keller. She became deaf as well as blind before she was two years old but lived a full enough life – as a pioneer educator in this field as well as an all-round human being – until she was eighty-eight. Her wisdom has not dated.

Certainly, when you have hearing loss, whispering, for a start, becomes a thing of the past, and you realize that from now on you will have to make do without the treasured (in retrospect) little asides you would make to your neighbour or your neighbour would make to you as you sat together at a lecture, in a concert hall or theatre or at any social gathering. The same goes for the impromptu exchanges with the person you pass in the street, or the assistant in the shop, or the barman, or bus conductor – or anyone anywhere. They might as well no longer take place. You have to make do with a wan smile and the realization that nothing you hear can any longer be taken for granted.

The pain that may be induced by an awareness of the accumulation of these little losses can catch you unprepared and you can even find it intense. The person you are with – in a café, on public transport or even in your own or somebody else's sitting-room – says something to you, a single sentence perhaps, off the cuff. You lean forward, anxious to hear and respond, say 'Sorry' and ask them to repeat what they have just said, to which they then say, unthinking, 'Never mind' or 'Oh, it doesn't matter' and – often with a friendly smile – make a gesture with their hand which seems, however good-naturedly, to be brushing the thought, and possibly you, off the agenda.

However, the pages that follow are not intended as an exercise in self-laceration, although I do unashamedly spell out some of the feelings that hearing loss has forced upon me. This is partly because I have been reassured to learn in the last few years that I am by no means alone, and that many, many others – who have often had what used to be called 'standing' in the circles they moved in, the respect of their peers and even accomplishment in their lives and careers – have had or are having similar experiences. Perhaps that fact may come as something of a surprise. But if you ask otherwise perfectly normal, healthy people, as I have done, what has been the main impact of hearing loss on their lives, they almost invariably home in on the word 'isolation', quite often with the adjective 'devastating' placed in front of it. Otherwise, perfectly normal, healthy people . . .

One of the most beautiful pieces of music I have ever heard, before my hearing went, lives on in my mind, enhanced by the fact that I shall never hear its like again. It came when Angela and I were on a group holiday together in Egypt and we had paused on a bus trip for the usual reasons in the middle of the desert, about twenty or thirty miles out of Cairo. The trip was a good one, the group was in congenial mood, and there was an appropriately glorious sunset to mark the end of a long, hot and satisfying day. We were all quietly contented as we stretched our legs.

As we smiled at one another, the way groups do when they don't need to say anything, we became aware of someone singing, somewhere out of sight. In a moment, we realized that they were men's voices, unaccompanied, full throated and with a marvellous sense of rhythm. Then we saw them. They were labourers returning from a building site somewhere over the horizon, going home to families in the city. There were about a dozen of them, all in colourful robes, squashed together as they stood in the back of a rather ramshackle pick-up truck, holding on to the struts of its rusting framework to keep themselves upright. And they were singing for all they were worth.

From being a quiet and barely distinguishable, but insistent, sound on the horizon, their voices had swelled as they approached, reaching a sort of crescendo as the men passed, waving to us and grinning as they went, but singing all the way. Magically, it seemed, as they set off in pursuit of the setting sun, their voices grew quieter. And the silence of the desert returned. But as an experience from one of my last clear hearing days those moments will always be treasured and, in a secret bolt-hole of my mind, will be replayed from time to time, like a favourite CD or – remember them? – a gramophone record. The incident now has the same special preciousness as a tiny statuette I bought in a roadside café in Vietnam made out of bits of discarded Coca-Cola tins or, rather more grisly perhaps, the chunky piece of rusty barbed wire which I picked up on a First World War battlefield by the River Somme.

I gave an account of that musical experience in one of the most difficult pieces I ever had to write in twenty years as a journalist working on the *Guardian*. It was a very egocentric piece – me remembering hearing, me not hearing, me getting wistful about what was lost – but it drew more correspondence than almost anything else I wrote for the paper. At the urging of some who read it, it became a trigger for this book. Now, as this book has progressed to completion – and I always write the introduction last – I have decided I don't want it to be regarded as an exercise in gloom. Rather, I would like it to be seen, in a nutshell, as partly a chunk of nostalgist ranting for what has been taken from me but partly also as an examination of the feasibility of striking a sort of balance, of coping. In between, it will seek to offer some diversions – coach trips of the mind if you like – to look at the lives of a select handful of others who have been hearing impaired, to glimpse some of the highlights, and lowlights, in the history of attitudes to and treatments for hearing loss and to pause for a suppressed and angry smile at some of the blatantly fraudulent quackery of the solutions that have been offered, and in some places still are, to cure the condition. (The answer, before you consider taking up any such solutions, is to get expert advice – assuming it can be trusted!)

The conclusion of the book is that there is in fact more than one light at the end of the tunnel. There are ways, whether they are mechanical, medicinal or psychological, of coming to terms with hearing loss, and there may be some bafflement in deciding which way to go. But there is advice available, even if the experts dispensing it can be rather thin on the ground, and there are strategies that can be adopted. At the end of the longest day, therefore, there can be no doubt that living with the unwished-for loss (and not just of hearing) and the concomitant discomfort can be eased. Even the toughest mountains can be climbed.

Every writer puts down their pen or (in my case) closes his laptop with a list of acknowledgements and thanks, aimed at people who have been invaluable supports in time of need, or who have given essential help, or have been patient, or have simply been around, during the writing process. On this occasion, any list is bound to be incomplete. This has been in many ways the hardest book, out of a dozen or so, that I have written or edited. Teasing secrets out of practising Communists – who provided me with intriguing source material and a fascinating career when I did real work for a living – was often easier than quantifying what I could or could not accept as gospel from people with or working with hearing loss. It is a fraught and complicated and often spikily political area.

But I willingly acknowledge the help and guidance given by a number of individuals at the Royal National Institute for Deaf People (RNID) and its many branches and departments, and especially the always good-natured Mary Blackett and staff at the RNID library, and Dawn Dimond, magnanimous friend and sometime editor of the institute's magazine *One in Seven*. The RNID, as I note in passing, is more than a charity, it is a vibrant community, a society even, with its own sub-groups and its own code of behaviour. In addition, among many, I would single out John Ballantyne, a widely respected audiologist, who meticulously read the manuscript for me and offered guidance in several sensitive areas; and Michael Buckingham, a fellow lip-reader and one-time academic, as well as the meticulous Jim Pitt, who did the same. They offered corrections and amendments which I have incorporated as zealously as I could – although, of course, any remaining errors are mine.

There was also guidance from some distinguished but discreet individuals who have played a key role in the planning of the new Centre for Auditory Research at London's King's Cross; the teams at Defeating Deafness and especially Vivienne Michael and Geraldine Oliver; at Hearing Concern, where Fiona Robertson and staff were always unstintingly helpful; and at the Link Centre, down at Eastbourne, where Katarina Sherbourne and colleagues provided a welcome cup of tea when it was most needed. The UK Council on Deafness was also particularly helpful; and Barrie Porter, as ever, kept my head above water when computer technology became baffling.

I would like, as always but also especially seriously, to thank my wife Angela for allowing, with as good a temper as she could muster, yet more infringements into our retirement time. And I would like particularly to dedicate the whole of the book to the lip-reading group and Jane Williams, their teacher, who, since the autumn of 2003, have allowed me to join them for two hours every Wednesday morning in a rather bare south London schoolroom. From them I have learned that lip-reading can be very baffling for the first few years, that life has some very serious moments but also some moments that are deliciously heart-warming and funny, even when you have an invisible disability. This group has taught me that there is life after loss and, for that reason, that is precisely what this book is all about.

MICHAEL SIMMONS
London and Tideswell
2004

ONE

Into a tunnel

OLD QUESTIONS PERSIST, yielding perennially unsatisfactory answers: What is it in the human psyche that makes us slow down on the motorway to look at the debris of a crash on the other side, sometimes lingering to such an extent we nearly cause another crash on our own side? What is it that draws us into a little knot of spectators if someone collapses on the pavement or starts a noisy fight with a neighbour? Or, on another tack, what is it that makes us withdraw in confusion when a dishevelled homeless person asks if we can spare any change and what, apart from economic circumstances, makes so many of us hesitate, if only for a moment, when we throw into the bin yet another begging letter from a reputable charity?

At arm's length we seem willing to demonstrate a great deal of sympathy for the less well off, whether they are earthquake victims or those whom we see on television screens scavenging on the rubbish dumps in a poor country or those who may be blind or otherwise disabled and experiencing difficulty in crossing the road. Many charities for the less than privileged do very nicely from the sale of greetings cards – a convenient and relatively painless way of giving – but many remain desperately short of money and may lack the volunteer staff they always need for the job in hand.

We sympathize when we walk or drive past a queue on the pavement waiting for a bus because the one they started out on has broken down or, a more familiar situation, because there are repairs being done on the nearby railway line and there just aren't any trains. Poor unfortunates, we may think. And if it's the passengers from a packed double-decker bus who are waiting there, we would doubtless sympathize all the more if some of them were maimed in some way or on crutches or had an arm in a sling, their neck in a brace or were sitting in a wheelchair.

These would be the visibly unfortunate. Their situation is immediately understood. But what about the millions – yes, millions – who are in comparable circumstances but whose misfortune is invisible?

People who are deaf, including the congenitally affected, the completely deaf and the profoundly deaf, together with those who have a degree (mild or severe) of hearing loss, all have a condition – in some cases a disability – which is actually invisible. Together, they constitute at least one in seven of the population. Almost everyone in the population, I have read, is touched at some point in their lives by what is euphemistically called 'hearing impairment', in themselves or in a close relative or friend, for it is the most common sensory disability in the developed world. Defeating Deafness, a hearing-research funding organization, has found that ear problems account for one in every three visits to the doctor in the first eighteen months of a person's life and also that four out of every five pre-school age children suffer from glue ear. After childhood the causes of deafness and hearing loss multiply inexorably, at work and at play, and I shall discuss some of them in detail in later pages. But the stark truth of the bottom line is that more than half of the over-sixties in Britain today are deaf or hard of hearing.

However, because it is a disability which usually cannot be seen, those with hearing loss who may be standing in the bus queue or anywhere else may appear at first sight to belong with the rest of us. But now, picture these people, if you will, in a picture painted by one of those artists of another era who seemed to spend so much of their time depicting freaks and monsters. Why not exchange those who are deaf-but-don't-show-it with the visibly lame, the injured, the blind and so on? If you do this, pretty quickly you end up with something barely comprehensible and barely digestible.

Perhaps you will say this is a grotesque way of depicting hearing loss, and some readers may reject the analogy as unacceptable; others who really know will confirm that it is one way of underlining an inescapable statistical fact. It is not a comfortable piece of imagining, and it is not intended to be, but it is not without a measure of validity. Some individuals who are newly affected by deafness or hearing loss insist that they are in no way disabled and they are quite capable of looking after themselves, thank you very much, but others talk openly and even angrily of mourning what has gone and of the isolation that has come to them as a result. They argue that there are no acceptable euphemisms in their part of the world. They know that of course technology may help, but it does not – and cannot – cure.

It is important to mark out some of the essential differences between complete or near-complete deafness and age-related hearing loss. The latter is, of course, a form of deafness, but the differences between this lesser extent of loss and the fuller loss are at the same time simple and hugely complicated. When you are or you become completely deaf, you know you have entered into and remain enclosed in a more or less separate world, and, although you may sometimes be intensely lonely, you may also have grown used to living life for twenty-four hours a day without hearing. You have little choice, in fact. Scientists and others, on the other hand, have argued that some deaf people generally make better adjustments than those who become hard of hearing. Even if, at a comparatively early age, you have been obliged, as the composer Beethoven put it, to become 'a sort of philosopher', you know there are steps that you can take to retrieve something of a life worth living and that, if you are lucky, you can find yourself part of a familiar peer group. There are deaf schools and social centres just as there are clinicians, technicians and academics in innumerable centres who have some confidence in their specialist knowledge of the deafness problem.

With age-related hearing loss, on the other hand, only some of these resources may be available or appropriate. You are, in fact, in a very different category. It is not improbable that you will see yourself, often at a very vulnerable age, as someone who has been cast adrift on a wide, wide sea with no familiar landfall in sight. You have been a social, hearing animal all your life, possibly with some distinction in your chosen sphere of activity, and then, suddenly, you find this strange and gnawing loneliness has been thrust upon you. A moment may come – and I have lived through such moments – when you feel snubbed by the people who are sitting at the same table, when they quite blatantly and thoughtlessly ignore you, forgetting the fact that you just can't participate because you are not hearing what is being said. You are summarily cut off from the life you knew, and now you don't know how to react.

Until such a time you may have thought of hearing loss as something other people make jokes about. Perhaps you have made such jokes yourself. So now, how should you behave? Should you shrink inside your clothes, should you be ashamed, or not? Should you perhaps try to make the best of it? But how? Where are the rules? Should you adopt a phoney nonchalance, conveyed through a brittle smile, and announce to all and sundry, 'Oh, it's nothing really', knowing as you say it that you're lying through your teeth?

It goes without saying that the totally deaf are in many ways wretchedly disadvantaged, socially, culturally, professionally and educationally. But they do, in fact, belong, if they are outgoing enough, to a vigorously defined group that has its own integrity and its own standards and norms. Men and women who have come to age-related hearing loss in late middle age, on the other hand, are barely acquainted with such a clearly defined integrity. Obviously one has to avoid anomalous generalizations, but individuals with hearing loss, although they are happy enough participating in small groups, tend nevertheless to feel disoriented in the much larger, but barely defined, group that runs into millions and which seems to lack any serious coherence. For these individuals, life from now on is likely to be more about avoidance than about convergence.

Exclusiveness and unashamed assertiveness are twin planks of the platform from which deaf people are able to argue their case. When you meet a lot of them together, as I have done on numerous occasions since losing my hearing more than half-a-dozen years ago, you can be bowled over by the animation and sometimes sheer exuberance with which their representative talk to each other and anyone interested in their cause. Deaf fairs, which are held up and down the country and are attended by hundreds of hearing-impaired folk every day of their run, can have all the bewildering medley of sound – and unadulterated noise! – that one associates with fairs of any sort. There are people busy buying and selling, shouting the odds for their interest group and, always, excitedly talking and talking – either orally or through sign language – to each other. The first one that I visited was, as the deaf themselves would be the first to admit, and like most of the others before or since, a world that was different from any that I had previously experienced.

At the spacious but crowded offices of the Royal National Institute for

Deaf People (RNID), in an otherwise quiet back street just beyond the boundaries of the City of London, there is the same sense of latent excitement in the air. At the RNID hearing people and people with little or no hearing work side by side, pursuing a whole range of different activities. As you see the staff members walking across the floor of one of their open-plan offices you cannot escape the feeling that things of unfathomable significance are capable of being discussed or planned. The RNID makes no bones that it is a campaigning organization and fulfils that role with a very assertive flair. But it is also highly proactive as a doing organization. Its activists and its fundraisers, its publicists, those who produce its glossy publications, its researchers, its spokespeople seem all to be full of a vitality and sense of purpose that other, more ordinary charities must envy.

The reason is not hard to find. It comes back to the controversial fact that deaf and deafened people have their own clearly defined culture, their own codes, their own expectations and, most important, they are generally able to support each other – to the hilt – in their endeavours to see these expectations, large or small, fulfilled. There may be fewer deaf clubs than there used to be, for a variety of often extraneous reasons, but still the welcome-to-the-club attitude when a newcomer comes along seeking membership of a local deaf community is usually warm and genuine. I have heard, first hand, of a mother taking her new-born (deaf) child along to the local deaf club where there was unalloyed joy, not just at the thrill of greeting a new baby but also at the prospect of another individual person adding to the solidarity of their cause. I have also heard that the local deaf club in one northern city is one of the noisiest places to go, which is a touch ironic when you consider that hearing loss caused by noise pollution is today three times higher than it was a generation ago!

It is when you start picking over the minutiae of their cause that the gritty assertiveness of deaf people becomes apparent. It comes, in part, from a long history of having to defend their corner against often unscrupulous and not always detectable adversaries. For literally thousands of years deaf people and their immediate relatives, who have sought wherever possible to foster their interests, have been the subject of controversy and argument. Somewhere near the beginning of recorded time it was a matter of course that new-born babies who were found to be deaf were flung over the nearest cliff or tossed into the nearest fast-flowing river. As I shall show in later pages, the Ancient Egyptians did it, the 'civilized' Greeks did it and even the civically responsible Romans did it. Then there came a phase when they were allowed to live, but only after they had been dumped at the doors of supposedly sympathetic monasteries or convents. Here there was always the possibility that they would be taken in and, albeit often as an inferior species, looked after.

For centuries, as I also explain later, the deaf and dumb were simply not talked to or talked about, and they and also many of the hearing impaired have been regarded with hostility and superstition. Some very negative views propounded by the Greek philosopher Aristotle, who said there was little or no point in trying to communicate with people who could not hear, did not help the cause. Only religious dignitaries – including Muhammad and some Christian leaders, who had little moral choice in the matter – have taken a lead in meeting their real needs as sentient human beings. But to this day there is plenty of evidence that the word 'dumb' continues routinely to be used for someone whose actions seem stupid or incomprehensible, which in turn means that, to this day, hostility and superstition are still something the deaf and/or dumb may have to contend with.

Discrimination remains endemic, even if it is unconscious in the minds of its perpetrators, in almost all areas of human activity. It is apparent in the planning and design offices in which architects and others create public places where people like to meet socially, and it is apparent in the office block, shop, factory or college where the hearing impaired might turn up seeking to work or study. I have heard recently of a holiday company that refused to accept a booking from two deaf people on the grounds that, for health and safety reasons, they would have to have a hearing companion with them. However, when some very weighty protests came in on behalf of the couple, this particular company buckled and offered compensation and even agreed to have another look at the small print of its policies. It may be said in some breezy places that it is a 'blessing' for a deaf person to be alive in the twenty-first century. For many that is probably true, but for an unknown and very large number it is not, and there is a chill in that breeze.

Only within the last three or four hundred years has the social and medical condition of deafness begun to get the attention it deserves, with serious and capable minds probing and researching what might be the reason for deafness and what might be done to alleviate the disadvantages. After the Enlightenment there was a period, particularly in mainland Europe, when the deaf were taught to 'speak' and to perform their meticulously rehearsed oral responses to prepared questions in front of audiences, sometimes running into the hundreds, drawn from royalty and the aristocracy. When the performances went well, royal patronage – as well as some unscrupulous plagiarism of original ideas – could be assured. When performances went badly, as for instance when the performers fluffed their lines or came in on the wrong cue, scepticism would resurface and superstitious prejudice would once again take over.

It has only been in the last century, and especially in the last few decades as the practice of audiology has come into its own, that a new cohesiveness of approach seems to have come into play in discussions about treating deafness. The word audiology was first used only comparatively recently, and a great deal of virgin soil has still to be upturned. But a bright new Centre for Auditory Research, part of the University College Ear Institute, has just opened its doors in London. The hostility and superstition may have been dissipated – although many think it has not – but among people who should know better, from legislators to opinion formers and from one group of researchers to another, there is still plenty of room for disagreement.

The arguments which have raged intermittently over the viability of sign language are a case in point. At a notorious conference held in Milan in 1880 of deaf people's (mainly hearing) teachers and administrators a vote that it should be banned was carried. This act of rejection was a move which set the cause of deaf people back a hundred years. 'Everyone knows', said one well-satisfied delegate after the conference, 'that the deaf are inferior in all respects.' Only in very recent times has sign language begun to get the acceptability that so many are convinced it deserves. At another extreme there are the arguments, which can be particularly virulent even among deaf individuals themselves about, for instance, the use and the usefulness of in-the-ear cochlear implants, especially in small children. These are arguments that will not go away in the foreseeable future.

But, but, but ... this is not a book about deafness. It is about that form of deafness called age-related hearing loss, which comes to millions of people in later life and which is a very different thing from total deafness. Clearly the experiences of deaf people and of those who have worked tirelessly with and for them will be extensively drawn upon. This is because, in a number of very important ways – in clinical treatment, for example – we are all in the same boat, mooring, as it were, at the same clinic. The deaf can be counted in tens of thousands; in the next few years those with hearing loss will be approaching the 10 million mark, a million of whom, according to very recent research, seem to have inherited deleterious hearing-related genes from their mothers.

The book before you has been written by a non-technical but concerned individual who has what might loosely be called average hearing loss – not really deafness – who more often than not gets by with an average National Health Service hearing aid. This is one which involves a lump of hollow, moulded plastic inserted into the ear hole and a battery-powered hearing machine looped around the affected ear. Statistically speaking, oldies with hearing loss, in the same situation more or less as this writer, outnumber the deaf by one hundred and fifty to one, but, at the same time, they get only a tiny percentage of the attention that deaf people get.

Such oldies used to be catered for by an organization called the British Association for the Hard of Hearing, which would run charabanc holidays to the seaside for members, hold lip-reading championships and promote local competitions to find out who had the clearest 'speech'. It has now been superseded by Hearing Concern, a small London-based organization, working at a social level with many affiliated organizations to improve the lot of those with hearing loss. It has volunteers who do, in fact, still organize group outings to the seaside! But Hearing Concern is one among a great many. The UK Council on Deafness, which, with a minuscule staff, manages to hold an umbrella over all concerned organizations, likes to count its members and affiliates by the score, and it reports that the numbers are increasing by dozens every year.

To draw attention to the quantitively less active interest that is taken in those with hearing loss, compared with the amount taken in the deaf, is not done out of self-pity or grudge, although there is plenty of both to go around, but to draw attention to a matter of fact. This, if you like, is one of the prime motivations for the book: the seemingly overwhelming evidence that, in a number of key areas of treatment and rehabilitation, the hearing impaired (as well, it has to be admitted, as many deaf people) simply do not get a fair deal. I know that if I wanted I could, for less than a pound sterling, buy a badge to stick on my chest which says 'Hard of Hearing, Please Speak Clearly'. But I want a bit more than that.

Recently I wrote to a retired public service employee in her late seventies asking her to write down what she saw as the biggest disadvantage, apart from not hearing properly, of hearing loss. She had had a distinguished career and remained a strong character with a very brisk and confident air about her. Her reply came in unambiguous terms. 'Isolation and loneliness,' she declared, 'aggravated by people not understanding defective hearing. For example, not giving time and space to face a deafened person when speaking and not understanding the enormous difference between those born deaf, who have never heard speech, and those of us with speech who have become deafened . . .' The only advantage 'in my entire life', she added, was joining the right lip-reading class and meeting friendly and joyful people with the same problems. 'We can all joke together,' she said.

Writers on deafness – like the books, magazines and assorted research papers which they produce – are many and varied. The schools and colleges for the deaf, not to mention the dedicated Gallaudet University for the Deaf in Washington, DC, are listed in every educational handbook. Research into deafness, as many experts agree, has a long way to go; but the amount of intellectual energy which has been devoted to age-related hearing loss, while it may well be just as much in strictly informal terms as that devoted to deafness *per se*, has a long way further to go before it may be considered on equal terms.

Probably this fact, too, has a great deal to do with the notion that, like old age, it comes to so many of us – even though nobody seems seriously able to define the word old in this context, for the simple reason that many more people are living much longer than they used to, and hearing loss may well occur before the other symptoms commonly associated with ageing. Meanwhile, research is going on to enable those at risk of age-related hearing loss to be categorized, to identify avoidable lifestyles and to recommend appropriate treatments.

The reality for most people, however, is that hearing loss comes at roughly the same time as stiffness in the joints or hair loss or freckles on the back of our hands, and there is a grudging but widespread accep-tance of the truism that it is indeed neglected partly because it is invisible and therefore of less obvious consequence. There is also perhaps a supposition that many of the men and women who have it may be seen as members of one of life's awkward squads. But wherever you may apportion the blame (if that is the right word), the impression remains that people who are affected by acquired hearing loss, in the words of Dr Ruth Morgan-Jones in a study published in 2001, 'continue to be neglected and notoriously to suffer from long-term identity confusion'. Their situation, from the sociological and health points of view (to name but two), remains under-explored, partly because it is inadequately understood, but one consequence of this is that it is therefore inade-quately treated.

You do not need to be someone who works in the deaf or hard-of-hear-ing field to be able to define the quickly discernible differences between hard-of-hearing and deaf types. Hard-of-hearing men and women may well be individuals who have been competent, even skilled, at their job – something they started doing when they were hearing. Their problems have arisen when they started having difficulties communicating with unsuspecting, hearing colleagues. Deaf individuals, on the other hand, may have fewer problems communicating with each other, although they may have to sign or use interpreters to get them out of difficulties with those who can hear. But, clearly, they may obviously need more sup-port on the job than their hard-of-hearing mates.

In the summer 2003 issue of a specialist journal for lip-reading teachers called *Catchword* I read the thoughts of a columnist called Chris Martin, who said she had long ago reached the conclusion that acquired deafness could cause what she called 'paralysis of the personality'. She added, 'I don't think people with normal hearing can be fully aware of the impli-cations of acquired hearing loss. When your personality is paralysed, you may no longer function as a lively member of your society, any more than a physically paralysed person can step out confidently into his or her former world.' With great prescience and extraordinary sensitivity she hit an extremely important nail right on the head when she also pointed out, 'People with acquired deafness encounter more blows to their self-esteem and have fewer means of pulling themselves up again, than those who haven't experienced this loss.' There must be many hundreds of walls and notice-boards in many, many environments where that particular sentence could be very profitably displayed. (Perhaps some doctors' surgeries and some NHS audiology clinics would be interested!)

The British government of the day as I write has made some steps in the right direction – notably in pushing back further the frontiers which will bring an end to discrimination against the disabled – but it is routinely left to a number of charities, often of very slender means, to finance the relatively few research projects that are going on and to the dedicated few researchers to do what they can often on shoestring budgets. One of these charities, in its begging letter for support from the public, argues that a few donations in the region of £250 a year, the price of a modest desk perhaps, could help pay for a full-time researcher working on hearing loss. Meanwhile, despite the recent opening of the new Ear Institute in London – which incorporates the Centre for Auditory Research – there is still acknowledged to be a continuing shortage of audiologists. This means that too many NHS audiology units up and down the country are having to make do with underqualified people known as hearing assistants. It is a sad fact that, so far as those with acquired hearing loss are concerned, rehabilitation programmes, which were heartily endorsed by a government advisory committee more than twenty years ago, and which could clearly provide such a vital part of the healing process, are disconcertingly thin on the ground. There are some hearing therapists available – but you have to know where to find them.

I make no bones about discussing the stigma that is felt, usually privately but sometimes very publicly, by people who find themselves with acquired hearing loss. Perhaps they can only acknowledge to themselves what they feel – nothing unusual in that – but they may be more than a little sensitive about what they know of their inheritance. They may or may not know, for instance, that there was a time when those who were born deaf were automatically rejected or killed at birth. They may, perhaps, find it understandable when (hearing) people persist in making a bit of a very tired joke out of deafness, with hand-behind-the-ear mimicry and so on, but the joke is not always funny, by any means, to those who are suffering. When hearing people start to reject the hearing impaired, or the hearing impaired are obliged, in social terms, to reject themselves, the situation becomes even less funny. Despair, in one form or another, frequently sets in. Men, it seems, suffer more, statistically, than women in this regard from what I have seen in textbooks described as 'identity disruption'.

Deaf people, on the other hand, have a certain truculence about them. They seem able, in a very literal sense, to trumpet the fact that they are deaf. 'I am Deaf and proud of it' is the first challenging sentence in a very challenging and very recent book of essays on deafness, called *Deaf Identities*, edited by George Taylor and Anne Darby and published by Douglas McLean, a small but very efficient company in the West Country. Jennifer Dodds, the author of this first essay, says in conclusion, 'One thing I cannot stand is paternalism and the huge amount of control some hearing people have over deaf lives . . . I have been appalled by the amount of "do-gooding" I've witnessed by those who pity deaf people and want to "help" us. Deaf people do not need help! We are perfectly capable of doing whatever we want by ourselves.' Her resounding conclusion is that 'one day, we'll all bounce together, so far into the sky that the enemy won't be able to catch us'.

Such bright and seemingly irrepressible optimism can only be commended and fits in very nicely with the twenty-first-century taste in iconoclasm. But it is also something that comes in the wake of the view, broadly accepted until a generation or so ago, that deaf people were in fact maladjusted, psychologically unhealthy and even incurable. Even in the dark days, however, there were signs of a will to fight back, although some very peculiar tactics have been used. In the RNID library in London I came across a book published in the USA a little over a hundred years ago with the improbable title *Deafness and Cheerfulness*. The author, A.W. Jackson, conceded that in his particular experience deaf people had grievances as well as griefs and that they 'suffered directly from their infirmity and scarcely less from the treatment of those about them'. But, with what I would call a *Reader's Digest* sort of queasy cosiness, he added, 'The brook still laughs, the wind quires, the insects hum, the birds are songful, the daughter's glee is musical, the husband's bass is tender and the wife puts smiles into her tones. Only your tympanum is out of order.' Only?

Irrepressible optimism is not something that is so easily found among those with hearing loss. Last Christmas I circulated the men and women who made up the long-standing Wednesday morning lip-reading class with a one-page questionnaire. Wishing them well for the festive season, as we sipped a glass of wine together in the classroom, I asked them to answer for me, anonymously, the same questions that I had asked the lady quoted above. What they thought were the biggest disadvantages, apart from not hearing properly, of hearing loss. Then I asked them if they had come across any advantages and, finally, what were the biggest changes, seen as well as unseen, that hearing loss had brought to their lives. There was a poignant consistency about their replies.

One respondent was a retired academic who had held a senior position at one of the country's biggest universities. He spoke of feeling 'socially stigmatized', something which, he decided, was a 'posh' way of saying he spent a great deal of time 'feeling a fool'. As a result, his tendency in complicated social situations was to withdraw rather than be exposed. The advantages, he announced with a pale sort of mischievous smile, were very 'definite'. He had found that the words 'mow' and 'lawn' had moved, as he put it, beyond his perceptual range – especially when spoken by his wife. At the same time and more seriously, he added that the noisy urban environment had become less intrusive. Speaking of changes to his way of life he said he had to put great effort into not letting it handicap him, but he still tended to avoid public meetings and performances.

There was also a response from a former white-collar professional person. The biggest disadvantages, he said, were having to re-ask a question and/or giving an inappropriate answer and not being able to participate totally in meetings, for example, taking notes or taking the minutes. The biggest advantage was being able to ignore a comment or a question on the pretext of deafness. The biggest change he had found was having to attend closely to people speaking in order to avoid missing anything and the anxiety and stress that accompanied this process.

It was on this question that my straight-talking former public-service employee, quoted above, had been at her most succinct. If her words in reply could be inscribed on a brightly coloured lapel badge I think far fewer old people would be called grumpy than is now the case. 'The biggest changes', she replied, 'are that I am no longer able to go to the theatre, concerts, talks, clubs, social events or to enjoy plays on the television or radio, and I can't hear children talk or birds singing.'

One of my more voluble respondents was a lady called Phyllis, who was aged well over ninety. She told me that when she lost her hearing at the time of giving birth to her daughter she had been overtaken by a complete lack of confidence. 'This change of personality', she said, 'is to my mind the biggest and most devastating effect of hearing loss. Very few people have any idea how to speak to a hard-of-hearing person.' Phyllis's devastation lasted for several years until she chanced upon a lip-reading class and found herself among like minds. But it has not entirely gone away and probably never will. Even at her age she felt constrained to mention it.

Jim, tall and dignified at eighty-six (he wrote his age in with his signature!) and still happy to be a highly active steam railway fanatic, announced that he had been ten years with the same lip-reading teacher but still felt he would never be any good at it. However, he kept coming for the congenial company. Bill, who is just three weeks older than Jim and with whom he has an octogenarian sort of Morecambe-and-Wise relationship, which is a joy to behold, said there were many situations in which he found himself where his hearing aid did not really help. The consequence of this was that he was now on the look-out in every junk shop he visited to find an ear trumpet. 'I think', he said, 'I am old enough now to get away with it!'

It is thus clear that the solidarity, although very real, is very different in the hearing-loss community from that to be found among the deaf. There is an underlying insecurity and an unfamiliar sense of persisting uncertainty that should not belong with people, many of whom will have achieved remarkable things in their chosen careers and yet now feel that others treat them as idiots because of the condition with which they have been afflicted. Although there is undoubtedly a certain satisfaction to be among fellow-sufferers (in, for instance, the lip-reading class), there is in many cases an encroaching tentativeness, an ever-present inclination to isolationism and even to depression. I have come across several accounts of mature men and women being reduced almost to tears – of rage, resentment and helplessness – when they learn that they are condemned to wearing a hearing aid if they wish to continue communicating or of similar reactions when they first put the thing in and, most poignant of all, of them feeling obliged to shun the company even of friends and neighbours who have hitherto been perfectly congenial fellow citizens. This is disorientation on a very big scale. For there are literally millions of stressed men and women experiencing, every day, a sense of frustration and anger which they have never felt before.

TWO

The curse of the hot potato

IN THE BEGINNING it can be rough, very rough. For, make no mistake, to experience sudden hearing loss is to experience a curse. Whether it comes suddenly or, I would argue, gradually, the totally unscheduled theft and then the irretrievability of the whole range of sounds that you have grown used to, taken for granted and enjoyed all your life can be heart-breaking. The intruder is someone who bursts into the home that you have made of your life, with all the brutal subtlety of a burglar, and then proceeds to wreak havoc. For many the experience carries the elements of trauma. You may just possibly remain the same person afterwards, but more probably you will not. A substantial chunk of your capacity for dealing with life has been taken from you and, make no bones about it, you have to adjust.

Losing your hearing completely and suddenly can only be described as devastating; losing it gradually is not necessarily any easier. In almost every account of the individual's reaction the key word to describe the first impact is 'isolation' – and I make no apology for this word's frequent appearance in these pages. It was certainly used by Heather Jackson, chair of the National Association of Deafened People, when she described her first experiences of hearing loss in the magazine *Good Housekeeping* late in 2003. It was very traumatic, she said, when her husband and children came home and they all had to face the grisly fact that communication could only be achieved by writing things down. She felt as though she was living behind a glass wall. She wrote, 'Often I just stayed at home and hid. If I did go to the supermarket, I'd spend the whole time looking for people who might recognize me. If I saw someone I knew, I'd rush to the back of the shop and hide behind the trolleys with tears streaming down my face.'

Hearing impairment need not be as overwhelming as that, but it can feel like it to some of those who have newly acquired it. Perhaps, given the statistical size and potential growth of the problem, it could become a political issue, perhaps not. Certainly, it is argued, there are many organizations concerned with deafness and hearing loss who are making what a top audiologist has described to me as 'a lot of political noise'. It may, of course, be a variation of family politics, but then it may be considered facile in an amoral society of a bright new century, where politics and government seem to be more about the murk of politics than about the obligations of those in power, to see an everyday issue such as deafness or hearing loss as a hot potato. After all, it remains one that tends most of the time to be conspicuously and studiously ignored by policy-makers – although some government-appointed advisory committees have done good work! – and it generally remains the sort of thing that gets the attention of ministers once in a blue moon – and then before a very sparsely attended House of Commons.

I used to work there as a Parliamentary reporter and was present on several occasions when an earnest MP would raise a subject dear to his heart or to his constituents to be heard at the fag-end of a long day by a junior, often very tired, minister and, at most, half-a-dozen fellow back-benchers. This was the so-called Adjournment Debate, and there was something simultaneously sad and fatuous about the proceedings. This was the debating chamber of the great House of Commons, after all. But was it really, I asked myself, one of the highest legislative bodies in the land?

The truth of the matter remains that deafness and hearing loss do not constitute, in the early twenty-first century, an area of priority for the government of the day. A top and officially engaged civil servant told a conference I attended in early 2004 that the dedicated care and health workers present should accept that deafness in terms of the national agenda was 'quite low down' – in fact, he said, it was 'battling against relegation'. Nor was the prognosis very rosy. 'It is never going to be high on that agenda,' he added. 'I am sorry about that, but it is a fact that you have to face up to.' Then he went on, with a curiously inept sense of timing, to speak of the incidence of suicide among deaf people. Just a few months after he spoke, in June 2004, the first meeting took place of the newly formed All-Party Parliamentary Group on Deafness. It will be interesting to see what impact, if any, this committee makes on the wider world.

It is understandable that politicians and aspiring ministers, if their hearing goes, may choose to get out of front-line politics. Having done so, they may start a new life, campaigning for changes in the status quo, a semblance of justice, in attitudes to disability, and they demonstrate with the rest of us – even in exceptional cases leading the way – when a suitable occasion arises. But one wonders to what extent they are now able to bend the minister's ear as they did before. What, I find myself asking, is the name of the Minister for the Disabled who has direct responsibility for the welfare of the millions who are hearing impaired? How big is the share of his workload that is taken up by their problems?

There is no shortage of charitable organizations, large and small, who are doing what they can to improve the lot of the hearing impaired, and I discuss the vital work that some of them do in later pages. But, away from the ministerial office, a seriously contentious aspect of hearing loss is that it is, in a word, to all intents and purposes, ignored. If you don't have it, don't fret. When it is not ignored it, too, often gets the poor-relation treatment from those whom the NHS likes to call health providers. Deafness is treatable, sometimes in very sophisticated ways, but it is not curable; and the same goes for the hearing loss, which, as they always say so nicely, is age-related, normally beginning at about fifty. This provides the providers with an escape clause, because it means that it occurs, in most people, on that last downhill slope. It is seen as consistent with the general deterioration of bodily functions, a sign of approaching and inevitable decrepitude, coming at a time when the Grim Reaper is beginning to sharpen his scythe. Perhaps, for some – including some general practitioners – it is too late to be bothered.

Disabilities, almost by definition, bring a privately nurtured feeling of apartness and anguish to the person affected. Self-pity is not seen – by others – as an acceptable option, any more than taking off one's clothes and carrying an explicit banner down the local high street is acceptable. There are, you may be told, many worse afflictions than hearing loss, and that fact is indisputable. There are also degrees of hearing loss, from the profound to the relatively mild. But how many of these afflictions, one wonders, induce feelings of fear? According to one specialist, W.M. Hunt, speaking in 1944 to a symposium on progressive deafness – which was attended by assorted psychologists and psychoanalysts – these included,

'Fear of failure, fear of ridicule, fear of people, fear of new situations, chance encounters, sudden noises, imagined sounds; fear of being slighted, avoided, made conspicuous; these are but a handful.'

As well as some or all of such fears, and the isolation and the anguish, there is the usually unavoidable challenge of somehow learning to live with a loss which you never bargained for and at the same time to find a way, somehow, through totally uncharted territory. One learned view I have stumbled across asserts that the psychology of deafness is more to do with the individual than with the disability. 'The lost dream', says Hilde Schlesinger, writing in the early 1980s in a book called *Adjustment to Adult Hearing Loss*, 'matters more than the extent of the sensory loss.'

A psychiatrist called P.H. Knapp worked with men, individuals who had healthy personalities before they joined up, who had become deafened during the Second World War. Writing up his findings in 1948, in the journal *Psychosomatic Medicine* on what he called the emotional aspects of hearing loss, he listed five 'compensatory and neurotic defences' that were employed by deafened people:

Overcompensation: adopting an extrovert lifestyle and bonhomie, with great emphasis on talking, which, of course, presents no problem to the suddenly deafened and in addition alleviates the need to lip-read and understand the other person

Denial: an attempt to lead a lifestyle as before, making no attempt at adjustment

Retreat from society: many found that the problem of maintaining social interaction was so great that the effort was not worth it

Somatic complaints: the emergence by neurotic displacement of a range of physical complaints

Exploitation: the adoption of a badge of invalidism in order to gain and subsequently exploit sympathetic feelings in others.

A popular alternative, not discussed in polite society, is to cast oneself in the role of victim, to surrender to withdrawal, something which may be thought self-defeating because doing so makes one wonder why one feels discriminated against. (Although I have heard of small housing estates for the elderly where some residents never leave their homes, preferring, somehow, their own company because they feel that communication would be difficult, if not impossible, if they left their own front door.) Of course, clever disguises can be adopted, and most of us at some time have known someone who has been 'very brave' in putting up with this or that limitation on their way of life. But there is no going back. This disability is one which does not go away, even though, somehow or other, a means is found of accommodating it.

But then you can be tripped up in unpredictable ways. Travel, for instance, becomes more difficult than it was. Security checks at airports, as we have learned to live with threats of terrorism, have become more stringent, with even hearing aids treated as objects of suspicion. 'Access for hard-of-hearing people on planes, trains and at airports, ferry terminals, railway stations, etc., is deplorable,' a concerned reader wrote recently to an equally concerned magazine. 'Sometimes, it is the difference between catching or missing a train journey or a flight on time, depending on how well you can interpret the garbled message on the public-address system.'

When your hearing is in order it is probable you give little thought to the quality of the public-address systems in your life. But then think of it in the context of an ultimate terror alert, which may or may not be upon us. If that alert is to be announced, as it were, through the loudspeakers, and it really is a case of the apocalypse now and 'Get out of here as fast as you can', and if, however hard you try, you cannot comprehend a single word because of the distortions, personal and mechanical, what then . . . ?

My cousin, Alex Jeffries, who is one of my best friends, wrote to me when he knew this book was under way, wanting me to know how he felt about his hearing impairment. He told me, 'I am secretly relieved that I do not have to endure the tumult of sound which is the lot of people with full hearing. I am told by those who should know that the computer inside our heads adjusts the incoming decibels to an acceptable level. I am suspicious of that theory and not prepared to wait however long it takes for my computer to decide what to do . . . I have therefore decided to live in relative peace and to ask my friends to endure the annoyance of having to repeat what they have said LOUDER. The only real embarrassment is when I miss the point of a joke and laugh at the wrong time.'

A woman who lives near me survives with the appalling reality that her legs seem no longer to be serviceable. But she still trundles along each morning in her mechanical self-drive chair to the local coffee bar, where she heaves herself out to sit in a proper chair and sip – outside if it's fine – and watch the world go by. Her small dog takes her place in the mechanical chair, alert and equally watchful. She seems to be at ease with herself, smiles at passers-by and talks with those who stop to pass the time of day. Hers is not – not visibly at any rate – a life of anguish. Perhaps it is one of sanitized anguish. (One sunny morning I told this woman I was writing this book and that I would be mentioning her, and she spontaneously reacted by saying she could think of nothing worse than losing your hearing.)

Doubtless there are some who put the same brave face on hearing loss, shrugging their shoulders and saying something like 'Well, that's life, isn't it? What can you expect when you get older?' A hearing-impaired psychologist told me that he thought it was quite possible that some individuals with an introvert disposition might even welcome hearing loss because it meant they would have to engage less with what they construe as a rather tiresome world. Where the potentially angry person might rail against having hearing loss foisted upon him, the introverted individual might go so far as to argue in favour of resigned acceptance.

Researchers have found that people with hearing loss tend, as a species, to suffer in silence and, although the number of hearing-loss consultations are going up sharply year on year, they still take an average of six months to seek the necessary medical help. They orchestrate their lives with a show of ostensible toleration, punctuated by a barely convincing smile or two along the way. A lot of us in this situation, I suspect, have no difficulty in turning grumpy and resentful and sliding selfishly into cantankerousness and bouts of anti-social behaviour. How else do we actually acknowledge that we are enduring times of uncontrollable discomfort?

Others are lucky to be able to rise serenely above it all. Nelson Mandela, who has coped with more setbacks than most in his extraordinary life, is apparently one of these. He has been able, publicly at any rate, to make light of his deafness. The French president Jacques Chirac, on the other hand, was publicly chided in early 2004 for not even admitting that he had a serious hearing problem. The British comedian Eric Sykes became very deaf, lost much of his sight and had a quadruple bypass operation but remained, resolutely, a performing comedian.

Hearing loss is by far the most common of all disabilities, affecting approximately 150 times more people than are pre-lingually deaf. The statistics when you examine them closely are staggering, and the incidence is steadily growing. The proportion of Britain's population who are of pensionable age has now reached a point where it is about three times higher than it was fifty years ago. Research shows that well over 8 million people are or have been personally affected by some measure of hearing loss, which is one in seven – some say nearer one in six – of the population. Three out of every four of those affected are over seventy – which is hardly the most convenient time in life to cope with a new personal setback, let alone the complicated technology which may be required if the setback is to be competently dealt with.

It is said that about 2 million individuals in Britain today use hearing aids; but it is also said that there are two and possibly three times that number, and probably many more, who could use them but, for a variety of reasons, choose not to. A hearing aid may be small enough to fit into the palm of your hand, but it is an extraordinarily tricky thing with which to form a balanced relationship. And one more statistic: the RNID help lines get seventy-five thousand calls a year for advice and information on how to cope with deafness and hearing loss or, roughly, one every two minutes of every working day. Scores of other hearing-concerned organizations, meanwhile, get thousands more.

The defined worlds of hearing loss and deafness provide, as they always have, a seventh-heaven situation for quacks and unscrupulous practitioners. For centuries there have been highly questionable men and women, sometimes parading trumped up or distorted qualifications from exotic and even non-existent institutions, who have sought to make their fortunes from supposed remedies, even cures, for hearing loss. One of the best known of these was the notorious murderer of the Edwardian era Dr Crippen, who, with a variety of non-existent partners, ran an organization calling itself the Aural Remedy Company from makeshift offices in London. The questionable quirks of the dealings of this company were something he seemed to get away with; it was the mysterious death of his unfortunate wife rather than his blatant quackery among the deaf that caught him out as he was sitting with his secretary heading in a westerly direction on a transatlantic liner. Fraudsters and quacks will be discussed in Chapter 5.

The commercial temptation to get into the pockets and purses of around 8 million quietly stoical sufferers must be enormous. Today's wool-pulling technicians – they are no longer doctors – have a ready-made and very needy market at their feet, reasoning no doubt that if only 1 per cent of those with hearing loss come forward for the treatment they prescribe they would constitute a ready-made queue of some 80,000 customers. And since desperation, depression and despair are the common characteristics controlling the actions of so many who are hard of hearing – individuals who might argue that any way out of an anguished situation is better than no way at all – then even 1 per cent of those 80,000 has the potential to provide quite a tidy income for the unscrupulous. It is hard not to be seduced by the patter, which comes, unasked, at regular intervals through your letter box and which promises, 'This could be the beginning of a big improvement in your hearing, and consequently your whole quality of life', complete with a freephone telephone number or 'The promise of clearer hearing' or even, simply, 'The world's finest hearing aids'.

The tragedy and the problems of those who have profound and less-than-profound deafness – when separated from those with hearing loss – are obviously serious enough, but they represent only a relatively small number of the total. Deaf children born to deaf parents have as much love and support as hearing children with hearing parents. The downside is the scandal and the hangover of prejudices which go back hundreds of years and result in the fact that so many of the congenitally or early deaf do not get the education they need and that they remain to all intents and purposes only semi-literate.

Those with hearing loss, and particularly with age-related hearing loss, are a stubbornly different kettle of fish. However, since their condition is not usually one they can flaunt or, however discreetly, advertise, it does not evoke the same level of interest or concern or even, one might say, the glamour, as other disabilities, sometimes including deafness. For technical and treatment purposes they do not belong to the deaf, even though they are not hearing in any satisfactory way. It is for this reason, among others, that, in relative terms, they are liable to be a barely understood species and, as even the specialists are willing to concede, their needs and services are among the most ignored educationally, sociologically and psychologically.

Overall, researchers have been willing to admit that the sociology of disabilities and of disabled people in general has been a neglected field. Within that spectrum the sociology of hearing-impaired individuals, and especially those who come to hearing loss later in their lives, is particularly badly served. The comparative invisibility of the condition is only one of the reasons for this. Another reason is one that comes from the accompanying sense of stigma that can confuse the thinking and the attitudes of the sufferer, something which may deter him or her from taking appropriate and cooperative steps that might help make life easier. The hearing impaired can be like the very poor, who come to feel that the act of getting the bull by the horns in an effort to remedy their situation can only draw attention to what they see as their shameful difficulties.

Of course, not everyone admits to the existence of the stigma. A few may not even be aware of it. Some are able, grudgingly or otherwise, to live with hearing loss, accepting it as the inevitable and constituent part of the ageing process that in many cases it is, cupping their hand behind the offending ear. A handful of individuals play the game of flaunting their disability. The writer Evelyn Waugh was such a person. When hearing loss came to him, he advertised the fact that he wanted an ear trumpet in the columns of *The Times* and was amused to get so many replies that he had several to choose from. He then made great play with the one which he eventually chose, disconcerting and sometimes offending eminent fellow-guests at dinner parties he attended, for instance, by ostentatiously laying the thing down on the table at the very moment they rose to speak.

The veteran Labour politician Tony Benn smilingly made light of his predicament when I wrote to him to ask about his experiences (see Chapter 6). in this as in other areas Tony Benn is an exceptional person. But, however you describe it and however well you adapt to its exigencies, hearing loss is a hardship and a bloody inconvenience. For me, being told for the first time by the audiologist that hearing loss in later years, like mine, was usually irreversible and could not be restored through any natural process – even though this was something I probably knew already – was like having a door slammed in my face. Some things, definable as well as indefinable, would never be the same again.

The anticipatory fear of being caught out by the loss is, not surprisingly, something that quietly haunts many people. But people don't like being haunted, and some go along strange and unfrequented paths, often pointlessly, in their search for preventive measures. My mother's favourite cookbook, which reached its fifteenth edition in 1928, offered a household remedy for earache: 'Put a few drops of warm olive oil in the ear', it says in a chapter called 'Hints for Mothers', 'and cover over with cotton wool or hot flannel. This remedy has been tried and gives instant relief.' In the previous century Charles Dickens, consummate exhibitionist and survivor as well as author, acknowledged that he, too, had worries about earache – and had his own way of dealing with it. It is well known that he would often walk many miles – in all weathers – to keep appointments. On one occasion, after some hours walking in the rain, he grew alarmed as his ear began to bother him and become inflamed – a condition he decided to treat with compresses of poppies which he held against the affected area. Then, being Dickens, he strode on.

We are not all exhibitionists and we are not all willing to succumb to homespun remedies. A much more common, almost normal, reaction among people with covertly suspected hearing loss is a determination not to be found out. Like Heather Jackson writing in *Good Housekeeping* they will take active steps to avoid encounters with other people, including erstwhile friends. I have heard in confidence and not a little astonishment from some individuals, whom hitherto I had thought spent their lives socially at ease with themselves, how they have turned and walked the other way or how they have deliberately – and unnecessarily – crossed the road to avoid the unpredictable inconvenience of having to talk with the person coming towards them. In such a context even friends can become an imagined burden, and some of them may be guilty of taking evasive action.

Lord Ashley – who was Jack Ashley, MP, and on the brink of a promising career when he became deaf – has written extensively and movingly on his condition. He reported soon after it happened that he lost none of his friends when he lost his hearing – 'but it was not until I was deaf that

I knew who were my friends'. Some people, he found, suddenly started gazing into the middle distance as they approached him and walked past him; others seemed with unexpected suddenness to become aware of the time and of the urgency of other appointments. In other words, some difficulty in communication was being anticipated, but the disturbing truth, Ashley decided (with remarkable self-control), was that while some conditions, such as blindness, may evoke sympathy, deafness is one that can evoke irritation.

Losing your hearing cuts you off from everyday exchanges, and you soon wake up to the fact that in losing even the most trivial of them you can be losing something that is strangely precious. Then, more to the point, the bigger sounds of every day become confusing. You become less aware, for instance, of the distance of traffic noise, and you may find it difficult to determine where this or that noise – of a motor car, for instance – is coming from. Thus, the danger of being run over as you cross the road is alarmingly increased. Even in your own home there is a whole range of new problems lurking. If you don't have an appropriate device fitted – and you may not even know such devices exist – you may be much less likely to hear the buzz of your own front door bell or the ring of the telephone. You may, furthermore, be even less able to hear what is being said to you by someone who is in the same room while, for instance, the washing machine is running its cycle or a noisy kettle is on the boil. One inevitable result is that even the most well-meaning relatives, friends and neighbours are inadvertently ignored or even shunned through an abrupt end to what has hitherto been routine interaction. The other result is that these individuals may also suffer as a consequence.

Less than an hour before sitting down to write these words I was on a London bus, opposite a woman who was clearly determined to make conversation with me. I wasn't really in the mood, but once she started it soon turned, perhaps fortuitously, into something of a monologue and I found that I was able to nod and smile at what seemed appropriate moments. She smiled pleasantly during our transactions and as she got off seemed satisfied enough. But I knew as I left the bus, much relieved and also with a tense feeling in the stomach, that I had not heard a single word of what she had said. I wonder if, in fact, she knew, too. Afterwards I reflected that I had in fact had a lucky escape: it could have been someone important and the exchanges could have been ones that mattered.

One answer in everyday situations like these would be to wear a badge, the way that some blind people do in Germany, where they announce their presence to the wider world with a yellow armband with black spots. For some hard-of-hearing people, even when they have acknowledged that their hearing is going, the decision to go for an aid is a very hard one – no decision, says the psychologist, is made without ambivalence. The wearing of the hearing aid itself, the equivalent for some people to wearing a badge, is something which makes them conspicuous but also perhaps, in an odd way, respectable enough. Badges are in fact obtainable (from an organization called Hearing Concern), but in the case of those who cannot shrug off the feeling that their hearing loss is some sort of stigma there is, once again, the question of who, to coin a phrase, wants to amplify a stigma?

One of the most difficult things to bear is the knowledge that you will be losing the little asides in normal conversational exchanges – the mortar, as it were, between the bricks of routine social interaction. Asking somebody to repeat the messages 'Nice day, isn't it?' or 'There's a fly on the window sill' not only destroys the spontaneity of the message itself: such asides may be trivial in themselves, but once you know they are lost, or thought to be lost, they take on a significance they did not seriously have in hearing days. My talkative woman fellow-traveller on the bus was joining, although she could not know it, an endless and steadily lengthening line: people in the street, publicans, postmen, shopkeepers, bus conductors, waiters in one's favourite eating place, usherettes in the cinema or the theatre and so on – all the men and women, and, sadly, children, as well (including my own grandchildren) – with whom little oddments of chatter have been part, and sometimes an important part, of the substance of the average day.

At the same time, you have, as the saying goes, to see the funny side of things. I went with a group of neighbours one evening to the town hall to lobby a local councillor about a controversial planning application. As we entered his room I asked if I might sit next to him as I had 'a bit of a hearing problem'. 'Not at all,' he said, adding, 'Down the corridor, first door on the left.' I demurred. Then he twigged. 'Sorry,' he said. 'I thought you said you had a urine problem.' Truly a dialogue of the quasi-deaf.

Many times while researching for this book I have come up against variations of the views propounded by Helen Keller, the deaf and blind American educational reformer who very succinctly made the point that is perhaps hardest of all to bear: that blindness cuts people off from things, but deafness cuts people off from people, from society itself. If you lose your hearing there is suddenly a whole range of people you regularly dealt with and of social events you would have thought nothing of attending who begin to fall off the agenda of familiarity. In a hundred different ways the routines of life, including those which can bring joy through the very fact that they are unrehearsed, are destroyed. The whole fabric of social interaction has been torn violently right down the middle. I have had many letters from grandparents who have quietly wept because they cannot hear the voices of their grandchildren. However many gadgets may be shoved into your ears or may be installed about the environment in which you live and work, no amount of clever needlework or tailoring or even of sophisticated technology can make good that tear in the fabric.

The symptoms of incipient hearing loss are easily described but far less easily acknowledged. Initially, without even realizing it, you may find yourself asking the person who is sitting next to you, or directly opposite, to repeat what they have just said. And then you may ask them again. Requests of this nature, imperceptibly maybe, become a habit and, slowly but surely, the unseen barometer of exasperation – something we all have, although happily we don't all use it – is brought into use. Your own barometer begins to give barely perceptible alarm signals when you find yourself thinking the other person has, quite unexpectedly, become somewhat incoherent they talk to you or that they have a strange speech defect – such as whistling through their teeth – which seems only now to have become evident.

I took early retirement from my career in journalism at the age of sixty-two. My wife is of the opinion that my hearing was going at least five years before that. But I was certainly lucky in my last employment, as I completed twenty years on my favourite newspaper, to be surrounded by some very tolerant colleagues who were not irritated when I asked them to repeat themselves and who, perhaps, were not able to acknowledge that they were aware of my problem. (A special belated thank you therefore to people like John, Victoria, Paul, at least two Davids and countless others for their forbearance, whether feigned or not.) I was also lucky in the sense that the hearing loss itself did not really get a controlling grip until after I retired. On the other hand, wearing a hearing aid in the intellectually macho surroundings of a hyperactive newspaper could have been difficult – for me if not for others. Wearing a hearing aid now when I accept invitations to social gatherings at that same newspaper does nothing to ease the pain of not hearing my old friends when I meet them. Occasionally I approach such gatherings with something approaching dread, only to be soothed on arrival by the very fact that these are friends.

Not only casual asides are lost, however. So, too, is the essential medium of whispering. This is something which we all indulge in much more frequently than we might think and which therefore assumes an unprecedented significance when the hearing goes. The person you are with in the theatre or at a concert or lecture very quietly confides an opinion to your ear about a moment that has just happened. But the ear isn't performing and, once again, you are in a position where you can't ask for a repeat of the message, and so an essential exchange is lost. A university lecturer, leading an extra-mural course I was attending as part of a London University extension programme, was so quiet that even when, with gentle ostentation, I moved to sit on the front row, it didn't help. Another lecturer I heard about from another friend with hearing loss was in the habit of dropping her voice at the end of sentences. If you are not careful in situations like this you may end up asking yourself why you bothered to attend the event in the first place or why you burdened your companion with your presence.

One of the obvious answers to the oblique question that hearing loss implies – one of hundreds, in fact – is that you have to get used, more or less, to living with a new self, which is another way of saying that when there are no other people around with whom to compare notes or to check what is going on or what could or should happen next you have to be strong enough to press on regardless. It is not always easy, not by any means. Some of the worst moments may occur when you momentarily forget yourself and the chastening reality that your own acoustics may present very real problems. Thus, you may arrive at the appointed venue for a business lunch or a night out – a restaurant or a place of entertainment – excited and anticipatory about what the next two or three hours may bring, until, that is, the waiter or the ticket office person asks your requirements or, worst of all, when your companion chooses to mutter a significant and confidential thought in your ear.

It is at that moment precisely that, metaphorically if not literally, you start to kick yourself black and blue when it dawns on you that for the rest of this ill-planned encounter you won't be able to hear anything clearly or the sounds that really matter will be distorted in some way. You don't know whether to feel stupid or sad. Titling in one form or another, or some sort of publicly provided assistance for the hard of hearing, as I shall discuss in later pages, is gradually coming to theatres and other public buildings near you, if only very gradually. But you can't get titling devices for a whisper from twelve inches away. As a general rule it remains the case that when an actor's word or a note of performance music suddenly seems unaccountably distorted it is in fact lost irrecoverably. Your immediate companion may of course be accommodating, but there is no way in which the actor or the performer can repeat themselves. They can't wait. They simply have to move on: most of the audience, after all, are hearing.

As you nurse the bruises accumulated from administering a self-kicking, you find yourself asking why on earth you bothered and how on earth can you apologize – yet again! – to the poor soul you have inveigled to join you? You are in a messy situation, where at least two semi-invisible barometers of exasperation are working simultaneously: one is your companion's, tactfully carried in a handbag or an inside pocket; the other is the one, not so easily concealed, that you yourself carry around with you. It is a fact of hearing impairment that exasperation – for yourself and whoever may be with you – is a constant companion.

So, what is to be done? Who or what can break down the invisible barriers? Answers are available but are valid only if, by a leap of the imagination, you are willing to assume that once the barrier is broken down the problem is solved. The NHS does its limited best, of course, but it can take weeks or even months to get to the head of the waiting list to be seen, even for a routine check. If you choose to bypass the NHS you have to spend a lot of money to be baffled with science and be equipped with a piece of apparatus you can't begin to understand. They may not all be unqualified practitioners out there, but there is a great deal of confidence trickery from so-called specialists and misplaced trust on the part of the inevitably gullible consumer. This is also something I shall examine in later pages.

Perhaps at school, when you were in your early teens and beginning to reason for yourself, your teacher set you to write an essay on the question: Would you rather be without sight or without hearing? When I was set this question, in the grammar school I attended in the north Yorkshire town of Scarborough, I was challenged and intrigued by the thoughts it threw up and wrestled for several days on how I might begin to tackle them. In fact, I do not remember sitting down to write this one (and I enjoyed essay writing enormously), perhaps because I had a cold or was off sick for some reason. I decided, without writing a word in my exercise book, that there is no wholly satisfactory answer. Perhaps this book is an extended version of that suppressed essay.

From the writings I have now been able to consult, by and about other people with hearing loss, the most widely accepted answer is that blind people tend to get more sympathy and to have much better treatment and services at their disposal than those with impaired hearing. The wider world seems to understand the predicament of poor eyesight more readily than poor hearing. Blindness is not a joke, and the white stick means serious business. Nobody mimics a blind person in the way that some individuals may laughingly cup their own hand to their ear and shout 'You what?' when talking for the first time to someone they know who has gone deaf. The campaigners at the RNID do not mince words. 'One of the biggest problems that deaf and hard-of-hearing people face', they argue with undiluted candour in one of their many leaflets, 'is other people's negative attitude towards them.'

On holiday in Glasgow my wife and I visited the School of Art in that city, an architectural gem in the career of Charles Rennie Mackintosh. On the top floor there was an exhibition of students' work – some of it fascinating, some rather outré and some beyond the pale. One exhibit consisted of a series of pithy sayings which had been written in blue felt tip on the windows – sometimes poetic and sometimes boringly prosaic – but always more interesting than they might have been because of the panorama of the city below which formed the backcloth to each of them. One inscription said simply, 'I wish I was deaf.' It intrigued me and I sought out the teacher and asked her to inquire of the student in question what on earth had made them write this particular sentence. She wrote down my name and address and assured me with the best will in the world that the student would get in touch. I heard nothing.

People with poor eyesight can now routinely go to their local chemist or drugstore or even the equivalent of Woolworths and buy a very adequate pair of glasses at an acceptable price over the counter. Even trained opticians have been constrained to concede that, judiciously selected and judiciously used, these specs need not be harmful. Certainly, for the outlay of comparatively little money the poorly sighted can quickly and conveniently find a way of resuming something approaching normal capabilities. The choice for the newly hearing impaired is in what might be called the opposite direction: you either have a tiresomely indefinite wait for an NHS appointment or you brace yourself, if you have the means, to spend hundreds, or even thousands, of pounds on a private device.

No such convenience shopping is available for people with poor hearing. A few branches in the bigger high street chemists are beginning to develop what they call hearing centres, but they have been unable to come up with any genuine bargain offers. Perhaps such centres are a thing of the future, although I suspect they will never be as plentiful as opticians. Boots, the chemists, in the shopping centre nearest to where I live – classified by researchers as one of the most well-off areas of the country – announces on its shop front that it combines the services of the pharmacist, the dentist, the optician and the chiropodist under one roof – no mention of ears or hearing (even though there *is* actually a hearing centre in this particular branch).

At the other end of this private scale there are the specialist hearing shops – usually small discreet places with friendly staff and complicated equipment and alluring posters of smiling people wearing hearing aids that, you are told, can be bought from well-known manufacturers. O brave new world . . . The first and, I hope, last such shop I visited, in a south London suburban high street, was courteous to the point of being friendly from the moment I stepped through its door. The shop was empty, no appointment was needed and one of its partners almost immediately became very solicitous, in a cosy way, to test my hearing capabilities.

After going through several hoops, trying on various appurtenances which were attached to my head and inserted into my ears, I finished up having a very amicable conversation with him – not on the latest hearing-aid technology but comparing notes on our respective experience of National Service. I finished up – no surprises here – paying the equivalent of three months' pension income for an all-embracing piece of moulded plastic containing electronic know-how, which, he told me, was carefully calibrated to meet the very specific needs of one of my ears.

The price, my fellow squaddie confided, was 'very reasonable', given the highly sophisticated technology involved, and, after all, I shouldn't ignore the fact that I was being given a special percentage token reduction because I was over sixty at the time of purchase. To an extent I really was lucky, and I could have parted with a lot more money. There are hearing aids on the market, I subsequently learned, which can swallow up the best part of a whole year's pension – and even some of these can be of highly questionable effectiveness from the hearer's point of view. But I had learned an important lesson in the pitfalls of gullibility when it comes to the private sector.

One of the big alleged advantages of my expensive new aid, the nice man told me, was that it could hardly be seen by the person I would be talking to. But even here there was a snag which soon became apparent: it meant, as I discovered pretty quickly, that, precisely because the person I was talking would not be able to see it, they would not, unless asked, adjust his or her speech to make it more clear. There could be no allowances for the hearing problem. Three months' pension money, I quickly decided, had been put to very doubtful use.

The choice until now has been, essentially, between free analogue aids on the NHS and supposedly more sophisticated aids from the private sector. The NHS's promise is that digital aids will be available for all who need them from early 2005. That remains to be seen. There is, at this writing, no approved middle route unless you count the disposable aids available at some chemists. For an outlay running into a few hundred pounds a time, rather than a thousand or more, you acquire an aid that will last a month or two before you throw it away and start again. However, given that your actual need will persist for more than a month or two, the outlay soon becomes much more than a few hundred. And remember, on decision day, that analogue aids make all sounds louder, while digital aids can tune out certain sounds while enhancing others. This means that personal needs and shortcomings, from the hearing point of view, should also theoretically be taken into account.

But there is a much greater hardship that is commonly acknowledged by all who wear almost any sort of hearing aid. It boils down to the fact that, unless one has a highly elaborate device – with a price tag to match – all sounds are magnified simultaneously. In any crowded room any- where, on any street which is busy with traffic and pedestrians, all sounds intrude intractably. Couple this with the fact it can be impossible to tell which direction many of the sounds, even those in friendly conversation, are coming from, and the result is what might be called aural pandemo- nium, with little chance of any lulls in the uncontrollable proceedings. One-to-one conversations in the open plan office, for example, or, if you are not working, in the supermarket, or any environment where more than one other person is present, have to compete with every other sur- rounding sound. Cinema and theatre foyers, I find, are invariably difficult areas; pubs and restaurants can be no-go areas; and television films with so-called background music can be non-starters. I am told that there is a phrase used in the audiology profession to describe the inability to hear clearly in a crowded room. It's called CPD, which stands for 'cocktail-party deafness'. More seriously, it is said that imbalances in hearing can be rec- tified by wearing a hearing aid in each ear.

So, at the end of the day, while it may be possible to adjust to loss, to come to terms with what has happened, it is rarely easy. A friend with hearing loss called Rosemary Lindsay wrote to me recently from south- east London at some fascinating length about how hearing loss had affected her experience of making music. 'I don't play the piano any more', she said, 'because the hearing aids I use have a very peculiar effect on the sound – all sorts of overtones twang and buzz and I have no idea whether the high notes are in tune or not. I still sing in a chamber choir that performs mainly unaccompanied music, but I fear that will soon become too difficult to continue.'

Then she added, 'I never would have thought that the noise made by eating would be a problem – with hearing aids, I find the racket in my head when consuming an apple or celery is overwhelming.'

When your hearing goes, you try, as soon as the initial trauma begins to subside, to resume, perhaps with the help of a gadget or two, a normal life. Only those directly concerned can know how hard you are trying. But there are no symptoms that visibly show that you are getting better and the adjustment can be very difficult. If you are living alone and feeling isolated with your new condition – a common phenomenon – the mountain can seem enormous and unclimbable. If you are trying to adjust while living with someone, and they say, unthinkingly and even perhaps meaning well, 'Oh, never mind' or 'It doesn't matter', when you ask them to repeat themselves, the loneliness is increased and can be piercing. On bad days an accompanying feeling of rejection can seep into one's consciousness. The brave face is not always achievable.

At the end of the day, there is an overwhelming and unavoidable piquancy about it all. The distressing fact is that you lose a great deal more than your hearing and the problem is much more than merely mechanical. You lose contact with people, with sounds, with words. This means that your responses, unavoidably, are also liable to change out of all recognition, and there seems to be very little you can do about it. The social, emotional and intellectual nature of your life, of Life itself, has changed. The old priorities and the old certainties, which all your life you have taken as read, can no longer be counted on.

Having written these words, I read that it is not politically correct to talk of the tragedy that is implicit in hearing loss. But, as Maggie Woolley, one of the bigger personalities at the RNID, has put it, in an account of how she became deaf while a student in Glasgow, losing your hearing is a tragedy. 'You have a right to grieve and to have your sense of loss taken seriously. You've a right to the best help and nothing less than total respect . . . [But] if you believe in life, then you must kiss the tragedy good-bye . . .' There is light, as I shall show in a later chapter, at the end of the tunnel, even if it cannot be greeted with that sort of exuberance. For the plain and inescapable fact is, you don't ever really leave the tunnel.

THREE

Listening to the silence

Entranced for a moment as I watch a flock of birds flying sound-lessly westwards in the limpid evening sunlight – without my hearing aid switched on – I find myself wondering whether we have per-haps lost the habit of silence. Ironically, it is a question you cannot help asking when hearing loss creeps up on you. Partly this is because, in your unfamiliar situation, you begin to appreciate that there are many differ-ent types of silence – those that are wished for, which may be treasured, those which may be punctuated by unidentifiable and shapeless sounds and those, often accompanied by an unquantifiable tension, that are not wished for. The latter could be called claustrophobic silences. There is no such thing, scientists say, as absolute silence. Even the blood in your eardrums makes a sound. Nevertheless, there is surely a range of silences which comes pretty close to being absolute.

Wished-for silences have a relationship with music. The seventeenth-century writer Sir Thomas Browne wrote of the music of the spheres, something he deduced followed logically from the supposition that 'there is music wherever there is a harmony, order or proportion'. An allu-sion, surely, to a very particular sort of silence. In recent years, composers – serious and solemn as well as popular – have sought to orchestrate silence. The extraordinary American composer John Cage declared that 'the composer must give up the desire to control sound, clear his mind of music, and set about discovering means to let sounds be themselves.' He also declared that if you 'listen to silence' it can very quickly become something 'deafeningly full of activity'.

Cage, who was described by an eminent contemporary as an 'inven-tor' of genius rather than a composer, claimed to have composed his most significant work, 4´33˝, halfway through his life, in 1952. This totally unscored piece was performed, and broadcast on television, in one of

London's biggest concert halls in January 2004 – 'a musical milestone', said the critics. Watching the performance, it was some relief that I did not have to adjust my hearing aid to accommodate what I heard. The only sounds were a cough or two, a sneeze and some not quite repressed laughter as the conductor, Lawrence Foster, mopped his brow from mock exertion at the end of the first of the three movements. It was an odd and beguiling experience.

Fifty years after the emergence of Cage's work the pop musician Mike Batt, who composed the original Wombles songs, was taken to court for plagiarism. He had produced a work of his own which he called *A Minute's Silence* and which, he claimed, was a 'much better' silence than Cage's for the simple reason that he had said in one minute what Cage could only say in 4´33˝. Although he finished up paying a six-figure sum to Cage's executors for breach of copyright, he said his first reaction to their claim had been one of 'hysterics' which only increased when his mother had asked him precisely which part of the silence he was alleged to have stolen.

Purposefully conceived silences may be wished for. At the other end of the spectrum are those that may be described as unwished for. One of these comes to me every morning, and is something I have never quite got used to. It envelopes me as I wake up, and no matter how much I strain, or how often I shake my muzzy head, or toss and turn for a few last fitful moments, it won't go away. It is not quite suffocating, although some might call it that, but it is – until I have inserted my hearing aid – totally pervasive, invading every corner and cranny of the room and the house. The hearing aid relieves it, of course, but the hearing aid is a device. This is one of the silences which is always there – acceptable in the night but disconcerting in the daytime. Definitely unwished for and even, in some instances, quite frightening.

It was the twentieth-century French writer Albert Camus who argued very cogently, and in a very different context, against what he called the 'unreasonable silence of the world'. For him this was a philosophical concept, one which had to do with the challenges facing an individual's search for identity in an intractable universe and nothing to do with deafness or hearing loss. But the anger that, however much it is repressed, may accompany the disorientation of the hearing impaired, is, in fact, comparable. The grim resentment that may surface as a direct consequence of hearing loss arises easily from what the affected individual may well decide is an 'unreasonable silence'. And all the more unreasonable because, henceforth, it will always be part of his or her life.

The unreasonableness varies in intensity because there are varying degrees of hearing loss. But it is always there, the muffled reminder of what has been taken away. If, in hearing times, you have enjoyed even the most humdrum conversation for its own sake or the sound of music or the theatre, or the incomprehensible interaction of twittering birds in the back garden – the list is endless – and if that enjoyment is abruptly and irrevocably curtailed and the involvement and/or participation to which it gave rise, then there are surely good grounds to think of that curtailment and the measure of silence that accompanies it in terms of the unreasonable. It can be thoroughly reasonable to be angry.

But if you suspend your anger, there is another side of the coin. This is that it is one of the fascinations of hearing loss that you have to negotiate, and then come to terms with, a whole range of silences. Not only do familiar sounds change in quality as well as quantity but the silences with which you were acquainted before the loss also transform into something quite unlike those which you knew so well before. With the best will in the world from the manufacturers, it is a technological fact that most of the hearing aids which have so far been devised still manage to distort, however minimally, the sounds which you are newly able to hear. This means that when there is a pause in the flow of the sounds, when something approaching quietness takes over, then that quietness may also not be quite what it seems. A different sort of magnification has taken place. This means in turn that it is impossible to define normal sounds any more.

Silences are things we have all grown up with. They become a regime, from the very moment our impatient parents or perhaps an early school teacher demanded that we should 'Be quiet!' when they were trying to read a newspaper or to keep order in the classroom, even though, in all innocence, we were merely being rather boisterous. When you're deaf, you go to the opposite extreme, perhaps to the extent of craving a little more variety of sound to break the quiet monotony that has taken over. Total or complete deafness brings an experience that only the totally deaf can try to quantify. According to one graphically described experience I have read about, there comes the new sensation of 'hushness'. Every day, this person said, it is like when you wake up in the morning and it has been snowing during the night and there are two feet of snow outside. Hushness is a magnification of silence.

Silences represent a pause, long or short, contrived or accidental, in the business of living. They can bring fear or they can bring exhilaration. Some have nothing to do with hearing loss but everything to do with the context in which they occur. The lull before a thunderstorm can be tense; the silence which may be called for from a large crowd, in remembrance of the recently dead, can be soothing; the pitch-black quiet of the night-time when you think there may be an intruder in your house can be deeply unsettling, and so on. In other words, quite apart from liking silences or not liking them, it matters also when and where they occur and, most significantly, whether or not they have been forced upon you.

For the hundreds of thousands of men and women who were active in the national labour force only a generation or so ago, when Britain was an industrial power, the silence which has come with enforced idleness has had an economic as well as a social impact. Where there was work, there was also noise. These people may have gone through officially benign processes of retraining and redeployment, but they have experienced a void, something that was unimaginable, even inexpressible, when they left school to become wage-earners. 'Noise', said an American writer, Walter Pitkin, writing in 1935, 'plainly shatters the ear, and the entire world has become bedlam . . . What a tragic absurdity, then, is our whole new and much touted economic revolution!'

Not every economic activity can be extrapolated in the same way, but for former dockers and shipyard workers living in or near the once great ports of, say, London, Liverpool, Manchester or Glasgow the silences along the waterside where they used to work must be eerie in the extreme. My great-grandfather, William Jeffries, worked on London docks until the middle of the nineteenth century. Then mechanization of some sort displaced the need for his manual labour and he was no longer needed. He died soon afterwards. On the Manchester Ship Canal today, where there was once frenetic activity as freight by the thousands of tonnes was loaded and unloaded throughout the year, there is now no activity, only the discreet bustle of office workers occupying the prestigious new office blocks by the water or the culture vultures who descend, especially at weekends, to visit state-of-the-art museums and art galleries in the vicinity. But then, along one fifty-metre stretch of the waterfront, you come across an eloquent but soundless reminder of the past. Sacks, barrels, handcarts and all the accoutrements of men working at the loading business have been, as it were, frozen static and painted a colourless grey. Even a pair of gloves is there, as if laid to one side just for a moment. This is modern sculpture, and it is strangely moving at first encounter. Its title, given on a metal plate, is *Silent Cargo*.

My own career as a journalist, when I was hearing well and using more than one language, took me for many years into the field of international politics and particularly East–West relations. It meant spending a lot of time in Eastern Europe, learning about the eloquence of (very extended) silence of a totally different sort, the one maintained with what could be called a truculent dignity by the intellectuals and dissidents whom I would meet for usually unattributable, and often very secret, briefings. The anonymity that they so frequently insisted upon was an aspect of silence, one which was not of their choosing but forced upon them by the circumstances in which they found themselves. These were conversations, as journalists like to say, that 'did not take place'. This was a silence of expediency, but it was one that carried a political message.

Invariably, when reading about the vagaries of one-party rule, whether in pre-Second World War Germany or Italy or in post-war Eastern Europe, it becomes clear that there were many occasions when dissidence, uncertainty and – every so often – an accompanying silence have, in one form or another, played an important part. Undoubtedly, there were also occasions when one side or the other, or both, would resort to what might be called a voluntary deafness – but that's a theme for another book rather than this one. Silences intrude in different ways . . .

'Tyrants', I read in my newspaper in mid-2003, 'are involved with silence as a form of control . . . It is where the words end, or can't go, that abuse takes place, whether it's racial harassment, bullying, neglect or sexual violence. Silence, then, like darkness, carries something important about who the authorities want others to be, something important about the nature of authority itself, and the way it wants to dehumanize others in the silence.'

Hanif Kureishi, who wrote this, is a novelist who, by definition, lives by his skill in communicating through words. His argument in this piece prompted the thought that, as the only animals with the power of speech, we should in fact be revelling in our ability to challenge the forces that would try to silence us, whatever the consequences. That is a brave assertion, although it is too late to put the matter to my old dissident friends in Eastern Europe. And how many hard-of-hearing people, one wonders, would know how to revel in the business of challenging the (unbeatable) forces who so frequently succeed in silencing them?

Sensitivity to silence and what it can signify can prompt different readings of even some of the most highly charged events in history. Sebastian Haffner, who became a seasoned commentator on German political developments in the twentieth century, was a law student in Berlin as the Nazis came to power in the 1930s. In his memoir of that period, called *Defying Hitler*, he describes very graphically an incident which disturbed his peace as he was working one morning in the lawyers' main library. 'As always,' he wrote, 'the high-ceilinged spacious room was filled with the inaudible electricity of many minds hard at work. The room was full of extreme silence, a silence filled with the high tension of deeply concentrated work. It was like a silent concert . . . No breath came in from the outside world . . .'

But it was a silence too implausible to last. He went on, 'Suddenly everybody raised their heads, and strained to hear what it was. The room was still utterly quiet: but the quality of the silence had changed. It was no longer the silence of concentrated work. It was filled with alarm and agitation. There was a clatter of footsteps outside in the corridor, the sound of rough boots on the stairs, then a distant indistinct din, shouts, doors banging . . . Somebody said, "They're throwing out the Jews," and a few others laughed . . . With a start I realized that there were Nazis working in this room. How strange . . .'

That was silence with an edge, one powerful enough to change the course of history. We do not all live our lives in such almost palpably fraught times, and few silences can have been as dramatic as that. But, as that extract shows, your perception of sound as well as silence, and your association of ideas with it, can take on many different meanings. In May 2004, with the imbroglio over the occupation of Iraq at its most intense, Tony Blair, the prime minister, was tellingly accused of 'sealing his fate' by failing to read the silence which can come even to a packed House of Commons. 'In Parliament', wrote Michael Portillo, a Tory veteran, 'silence is much more frightening than the din of baying back-benchers.' Blair, he added, instead of heeding the silence, plunged into 'obfuscation and slipperiness'.

When your hearing goes, your definitions of acceptable or unacceptable noise start to change. You expect hearing loss to mean what it says, namely the *de facto* removal or the blurring of distinct sounds and noises you have probably taken for granted all your life. But it is still strange in the mornings when, having removed your hearing aid, you get wet under the shower but cannot hear the flow of the water which soaks you, when you can barely hear yourself urinating into the lavatory or even the muffled sound of your own toothbrush at work on your teeth.

I couldn't help noticing that when I began scouring the shelves of the RNID library in north London the word itself shouted out to me its essential relevance for deaf and hard-of-hearing people. There were many, many books on its shelves, and especially those written by the deaf themselves, which had the word silence in their title – *Surviving in Silence*, *Children in Silence* and *My Sense of Silence* are just some (chosen at random) which are currently in print. The unambiguous message once again was that here was yet another whole range of silences – all valid, all different from one another and all suppressing the sounds that may, or may not, have gone before. Each author provided a different reading.

You are left with the option of pondering upon gradations of what remains audible and what has become inaudible when your hearing goes. To rephrase Shakespeare, some are born to silence, some achieve it and some have it thrust upon them. Not necessarily complete silence, of course, whatever that may mean, but enough of it to make a subdued, and subduing, contrast to the sounds which went before. It need not, by any means, be an altogether dispiriting experience, and sight should not be lost of the beginning of those particular lines from Shakespeare, 'Be not afraid of greatness' – or in this case silence.

I had a letter from one person who does not openly share such concerns and who, it seems, has remained grittily unafraid. 'Dear Mr Simmons,' wrote Lady Nicholson, a member of the European Parliament, when I asked her about her experiences, 'I was born severely deaf and with extremely poor eyesight. Probably both sensory perception deficits stem from my mother's serious rubella when she was carrying me. My life has not been hampered in any significant way – perhaps I work harder because I have to! Yours sincerely, Baroness Nicholson of Winterbourne.' No offence intended, but I could not avoid the feeling as I read it that I was looking at a political manifesto for a very moralizing political party!

Silence has to be qualified before it can be defined. Its range can be as appreciable as the range in tone and volume of the sounds it has displaced. In an interview given to the *Guardian* newspaper in October 2003 the Hungarian-born concert pianist András Schiff declared, 'I never play an encore. And I would prefer it ideally if there was no applause at the end, just a wonderful silence.' He was, I was told by a friend who attended one of his concerts (including encores), being economical with the truth. For some that sort of silence is congenial to the point of being almost magical. The twentieth-century Russian poet Anna Akhmatova, a formidable woman whose work chronicled, among much else, the siege of Leningrad in the Second World War, has told of the moment when, in 1961, after many years, she finally met the composer Dmitri Shostakovich, a similarly heroic figure. 'We sat in silence for twenty minutes,' she said. 'It was wonderful.'

During the Second World War the painter Graham Sutherland would, as an official war artist, visit the newly devastated sites of London to produce his celebrated so-called 'bombscapes'. Often, he noted, they were forbidden areas, which did not make his commission any easier. 'I was arrested several times,' he wrote afterwards, 'especially in the East End! Once there, I would look around. I will never forget those extraordinary first encounters: the silence, the absolute dead silence, except every now and again a thin tinkle of falling glass – a noise which reminded me of the music of Debussy.'

The silence that prevails, amid the inevitable anguish, immediately after a bomb has gone off may hold its own fascination, but a moment's reflection can bring home to the onlooker the irredeemable ugliness of what is seen. The same thinking – or should I say the same silent spasm? – may take hold of people in certain gatherings at the mention of the word terror, or when you are in close proximity to someone near to you who suddenly and unexpectedly dies. Or at the other, more mundane, extreme, listening, as it were, for the proverbial pin to drop or holding one's breath to stave off an attack of hiccups or waiting in a motionless traffic jam on the motorway. Pent-up irritation, or anger, like the gentle impatience of the musician (in a sound performance!) when someone coughs at precisely the wrong quiet moment, can bring their own sound and fury, however muted.

In the first phase, when you have just lost your hearing – a phase totally indefinable in terms of length – the unexpected sensations in the environment which passes for total noiselessness are many and varied. At the most rudimentary level you may panic for a split second or so and wonder if the battery on your hearing aid has failed (again!) or whether the device itself has reached the end of notionally guaranteed life or whether your own defective hearing has slipped yet another notch towards the dreaded nothingness. The ramifications are endless.

The novelist Muriel Spark has found her own way of talking about the substance of silence. 'So great was the noise during the day,' she wrote in a novel called *A Far Cry from Kensington* (1988), 'that I used to lie awake at night listening to the silence. Eventually, I fell asleep contented, filled with soundlessness, but while I was awake I enjoyed the experience of darkness, thought, memory, sweet anticipations. I heard the silence.' But then, when Spark was writing those words, government statisticians and others had already begun zealously to measure the encroachments of, for example, popular music, of high-powered traffic, of the pace of life (as depicted and characterized by strident newspaper headlines). The noise from these and many other sources has been intensifying steadily ever since – to choose a random date – the end of the Second World War. But although silence, as an area for reflective thought, may have gone out of fashion, the predatory impact of noise has been increasingly acknowledged.

Acts of Parliament have been passed to abate noise, and newspaper boffins have warned their readers that a great deal of modern music carries inherent dangers. 'A new report', declared one solemn note in a newspaper from May 2003, 'shows that many clubbers are risking early deafness by listening to music at dangerously high levels.' One in five of all young people are deliberately exposing themselves to what are scientifically seen as dangerous levels of noise pollution, and two out of every three gig-goers and clubbers are known to experience the symptoms of incipient hearing loss after a night out.

There are now three times as many young people exposed to potentially dangerous noise levels than there were a couple of decades ago, and the risks to their hearing in later life are correspondingly greater. But then, there cannot be many young people who would take ear plugs to a pop concert and who would take a break of, say, ten minutes every hour, to give the recommended respite to their besieged ears. One of the more ironical reasons for the stodgy image of deafness and hearing loss is that it has no appeal in an era where youth culture is the predominant theme. The Americans have an organization called HEAR (Hearing Education and Awareness for Rockers), dedicated to raising awareness about the dangers implicit in what it calls 'excessively loud sound levels' in music – whether playing or listening, even through earphones. In spring 2004 the Beatles' elder statesman Sir Paul McCartney was ordered to turn down the volume of his practice sessions at the Millennium Dome. People across the Thames on the Isle of Dogs had been flooding the local authority with complaints. McCartney, as a consequence, was banned from playing louder than ninety-two decibels.

But concern, and even a measure of altruism, remains. At London's Notting Hill Carnival in 2003 a leading Member of Parliament was to be found distributing ear plugs and warning-literature about hearing protection to revellers in the noisy streets. Meanwhile, a directive from the European Union has been introduced to protect orchestral musicians from the noise of their own instruments. The BBC already provides individually moulded ear plugs, at a price, for all players in its orchestras. Some of the players, interestingly, objected to such official munificence out of a fear that if they admitted defective hearing they might lose their jobs. But what, one wonders, does the EU directive mean for future performances of, say, Beethoven's *Choral* or Dvořák's *New World Symphony* or Tchaikovsky's *1812 Overture*?

Perhaps another European Union directive could be addressed to thhe management of London Underground. Researchers at University

College London have found that sound levels on some routes are louder than a pneumatic drill – so higher than the prescribed eighty-five decibel legal limit for noise in the workplace. Regular passengers, they suggested, should consider wearing ear protection. London Underground's reaction to this news was a shrug of the bureaucratic shoulders: it was aware of the problem, it said, but didn't think passengers would be affected.

Industrial noise, despite the artistic endeavours of the aforementioned Manchester sculptor, is one of the most intolerable and often intractable causes of hearing loss and is, theoretically, preventable. Many communities in Britain grew up with noise and pollution from the latter-day dark satanic mills in their immediate neighbourhood. Many of these mills – like the coal mines and the shipyards – have been dismantled in recent decades. But not all: residual problems, and residual attitudes, remain. In 2003 a family in Devon, who had complained of eight years of unacceptable noise from the neighbouring shipyard, won compensation after the intervention of the local government ombudsman. He had decided in the family's favour after an environmental health officer who visited the family home found that he was unable himself to hear for ten minutes because of the noise from grit-blasting in the yard which was taking place at the time of his visit. Families with homes near the country's biggest airports, even those who have invested in double-glazed windows, have not been so fortunate. Their battles continue.

Researchers have pinpointed a gender factor in actual or potential hearing loss. Men, they point out, are more inclined to like noisy motor cycles and cars than women and are more likely to join the army and to use guns than women are. They are also less likely to wear ear plugs. One recent survey in Australia found that three men out of four, but only one woman out of four, will be hearing impaired ten years from now as a result of noise. Individuals of either sex who are concerned by noise levels at work are officially encouraged to ask their employers to submit their premises to a formal noise assessment and to contact the Health and Safety Executive for guidance. What such a request may in many cases do to the worker–employer relationship does not bear too close a scrutiny. What is certain, however, is that much more research is required into the fact excessive noise can kill vital cells in the ear.

There are no two ways about hearing loss: however minimal it may be, it brings with it an unfamiliar sense of frustration, often tinged with exasperation. It is possible that this frustration can consume you completely and, try as you may, you may be unable to avoid it. Metaphorically, as the sounds elude you, you turn around and cast about, as if you were looking for a pair of lost spectacles that were in your hand only moments ago and are now nowhere to be found. The piquancy is that, however much you grope about, your listening antennae have changed; the sounds, like the spectacles are gone – but for ever. (The frustration and the exasperation, I need hardly add, are felt just as acutely by the people who live with you!)

The eighteenth-century poet Thomas Gray is little read nowadays, but in the words he composed in a country churchyard he was able to distil very precisely the nature of encroaching silence. 'All the air,' he wrote, 'a solemn stillness holds / Save where the beetle wheels his droning flight . . .' When your ears are failing, or have failed, you know very well what he is talking about, but you also know that the encroachment is complete when even the beetle cannot be heard: its erratic flight across your field of vision may be clear enough, but the strangeness of not even hearing its peculiar drone can be unsettling.

You could argue that there is a topography that notionally describes total silence and the sounds whose outlines become muffled before they also give way to it. The whole spreads before you like a mountain range. While in the foothills you may pick out the isolated sounds that you can still hear as you can pick out a mountain peak or a tree or some other feature of the landscape that now confronts you. But it may be at the very moment you are doing this that you may find yourself overwhelmed by a sense of the relentlessness of it all. The realization dawns that you have no choice but to take on board the barely palatable truth that your immediate environment – your personally perceived landscape – has changed for ever. From now on, when you may be about to say 'I see what you mean', meaning 'I hear what you say' or 'I understand', you have to think before you speak. This is because you may not, in fact, have heard the detail of what was said and therefore you don't see precisely, let alone hear, what was meant. Perception in a whole range of everyday areas has become a different process from what it was before. The substance of conversational exchanges has also changed, which means in many instances communication – and the relationships that grow from this communication – have also changed.

For the totally deaf there is no other world but the quietness and there is no way through the fog of its never-ending, unforgiving numbness. Of course, you may have learned to live with, even to accept, it all; you may still have a sense of humour. But even if, being deaf, you may feel inclined to voice a protest at the grotesque, one-sided unfairness of it all, you still won't be able to hear yourself speak.

Acclimatization is one thing: you can, it is said, get used to anything. That may be true, but every so often there comes the awareness of the suppressed anguish, even pain, which, as a deaf person or someone with profound hearing loss, you have somehow to learn to live with. On the other hand, when you are overtaken by some measure of hearing loss or so-called hearing impairment, at least you still have the capability of making out some sounds and you also have the recent memory of sound. Always, when you least wish it, there comes a reminder of the pain. 'There,' said my wife one sunny day, as we walked across some common land, not far from where we live. 'Surely, you can hear the birds singing now?'

'No,' I said.

Sometimes it can be an engaging pastime to differentiate between the silences one encounters. The piquancy of every one of them becomes very clear when you have impaired hearing. This fact was brought home to me as my wife and I walked up a Derbyshire dale, one bright and clear morning in early April. It was one of those welcome but tantalizing days, which, although bitterly cold, hinted that spring and the probability of warmth to come were not all that far off. There were no other walkers, no humans at all, to be seen. There were the two of us, there were a few sheep, some tiny new-born lambs and a few agitated birds. The rest was silence.

Any definition of even the most idyllic silence has to be qualified by the sounds that, once you sharpen your perception, manage to intrude. Another poet, William Wordsworth, on Calais Beach with an early girl-friend, ventured (in verse) to describe the all-pervasive silence as being 'quiet as a nun, breathless with adoration'. But then, he went on:

Listen, the mighty Being is awake
And doth with his eternal motion make
A sound like thunder – everlastingly.

So much for the illusion of supposedly pure silence.

So was it really silence that we met on our exclusive Derbyshire hillside? Of course it wasn't. A small stream trickled gently but insistently audible beside us as we climbed; the path we followed was littered with dead fern leaves and bracken which crackled sharply with every step we took; every so often, not far from us, a startled wild bird, perhaps a duck, would rear up from its hiding place in the long grass and fly off in panic with what seemed like a (relatively) noisy flutter; and then, far above us, but near enough to be heard, an occasional airliner, heading from mainland Europe in the direction of North America, would grumble its way across the clear blue sky, a vapour trail underlining its intrusiveness. Silence, in other words, is relative; it is in the unconsciously discriminating ear of the beholder.

There are any number of silences that you can hear quite clearly, whether they are punctuated or not. It remains reassuring that many of them are capable of casting their own sort of spell, even when you are wearing a hearing aid. The experience just described on the Derbyshire hillside was one of these. Another, which must be familiar to many people, is the one which comes every night, especially when for some reason you are unable to sleep. This is a time when there is, if you are lucky, an all-pervading stillness, even if it is one in which every unidentifiable creak or tapping sound in your own house or next door gives rise to fleeting concern, or bring comfort, depending on your situation.

In our particular situation, living as we do in a semi-detached Victorian house in a London suburb, we know that such sound may well come from our next door neighbour, who is a night owl of a man who doesn't ever seem to go (audibly) to bed until around 3 a.m. One night I woke at 1.30 a.m., alarmed by the disturbingly distinctive crackling sound of a blazing fire. I flung the curtains aside and panicked when I saw that the bottom of the garden seemed to be a mass of flames. My first impulse was to ring the fire brigade immediately, but then I thought (despite the hour!) to ring my neighbour since most of the drama seemed to be concentrated at the end of his garden. I sensed he was smiling a little as he coolly told me, presumably from a distance of approximately twenty feet – the other side of the party wall – that he routinely burned rubbish at this time to avoid the predictable complaints which came from his neighbours on the other side if he did so during the day!

It is one of the delights which define suburbia that there may be other creatures of the night. One night of dead quietness, as I turned over in my half-sleep, I was startled as the security light beneath our bedroom window suddenly came on. Once again, I leaped nervously out of bed and pulled back the curtain to get a sight of the intruder. It was a fox, who idly looked up and probably snorted at me as if I were the one who was intruding and then proceeded to stroll nonchalantly and soundlessly down the garden path away from the house. As I was willing myself to fall back into sleep, I heard its shrill bark – a reprisal of some sort for my disturbance of its privacy or perhaps an expression of slightly mocking impertinence.

Nor did the impertinence end there. The following morning the same fox returned, this time padding silently right into the house. It startled me this time because it advanced with a soundless and almost proprietary sense of dignity through the open french window, at least seven or eight metres into my fitted-carpet territory as I was about to settle in my sitting-room armchair with a cup of coffee and the daily crossword. It departed but took its time in doing so, only condescending to go when I somewhat stupidly, but not quietly, asked it to leave. (Afterwards, I reflected that, although neither of us spoke, there had been tacit communication between that fox and me. Words were not needed. It was almost a positive dialogue of the deaf!)

Such beguiling intrusions apart, there are other silences that can occur even in a built-up urban area in the twenty-first century and especially at night. They may have their own unfailing magic, which may even be enhanced for those with impaired hearing. Notionally, and most dramatically, these tend to occur when everyone else in the house is asleep and when you are perhaps on your way to the bathroom to fetch a glass of water or to relieve yourself. Nothing normally disturbs the stillness, except, in our case, the occasional creaking of a Victorian floorboard. It is a time when familiar objects become unrecognizable and somehow challenging, a time when an unquantifiable urge to explore takes over and when fantasies take shape.

The magic of a moment such as this can be spontaneously transformed if you look out of the window and you discover, not for the first time perhaps but always with a new sense of delight, the amazement of a full moon or, if it is high summer, that the sun is streaming down, even at four or five in the morning. These are moments when silence can be at its most pure, when very occasional night sounds, however muffled, serve only to enhance the silence. The plastic garden table and chairs, which have facilitated so many noisy meals and snacks during the day, are mute; the neighbour's cat, creeping up the path away from the house, makes no noise. At times like these, you may find that you are stunned into a euphoric wakefulness and feel oddly incredulous that this phenomenon called night comes around so frequently. You may even be grateful that you are not hearing anything, anything at all, just relishing the full the visual feast of everything, familiar and unfamiliar, that this full moon or the audacious sun is soundlessly offering, however fortuitously, and highlighting so magnanimously, with both arms extended.

Returning to sleep while such a feast is going on outside seems, even if fleetingly, to be out of the question, an almost criminal waste of opportunity. Small wonder that over the centuries poets have been stunned into writing so much about such things.

Of course there are other sorts of hushness, or near equivalents, and no doubt those who have pondered on such things have their own preferences. Some are more routine and more mundane, some are imbued with a certain undefinable atmosphere of expectation, even of tension. But only rarely are they complete silences. Public buildings, when they are purpose-built to accommodate hundreds, even thousands, of people at a time can be almost eerie when no one is present. An empty concert hall, football stadium, church, theatre or cinema, or even an empty factory floor or open-plan office can convey disquiet as well as quiet. As in a cemetery at twilight ghosts may be lurking: the quiet of the grave has its own momentum.

Evelyn Glennie is a very deaf but very accomplished musician, whose professional experiences are discussed in a later chapter. She has written of the 'burning, excited feeling' she has had in London's Festival Hall or the Barbican on those occasions when her fellow musicians had dispersed after rehearsal. 'I would often stay alone in the hall', she wrote, in her autobiography, 'after everyone had gone, to enjoy the silence and then the magical image of myself performing.' Glennie, incidentally, also told of tests she had had on her brain activity which indicated no response to speech but a reaction to musical sound. She resigned herself early on in her life to the reality that there would be no miraculous cure for her faulty hearing but then proceeded to make a brilliantly assertive career as a percussionist of international standing.

Even otherwise busy newspaper offices can provide havens for ghosts. I learned this on the odd occasion during my forty years as a professional journalist when, perhaps on a Saturday or Sunday morning, it became necessary for me to call in for something I needed very quickly, maybe for a piece I was writing at home, or for a trip I was about to make on the paper's behalf out of town or out of the country. Always, as I searched for my piece of paper or whatever, I found the lack of noise in a vast open-plan newsroom, which was usually filled with extreme agitation as weekday deadlines approached, was strange and uncanny.

Empty churches must be very refreshing spiritually for the church functionary or for the passing worshipper who similarly calls for something, spiritual or otherwise, that he or she may need, even if that something is a moment of uninterrupted contemplation. A friend who occupies an administrative position at Ripon Cathedral in Yorkshire tells me how he treasures those special moments in the early morning when he has the cathedral's silence all to himself. A vow of silence is the very essence of the life of the Trappist monk. And what about empty houses and especially big empty houses? Some of them somewhere must surely give some burglars a pause for thought. It is always possible that some intruders who perform their break-ins in the dead of night may find themselves subject to fleeting moments of what might loosely be called 'breaking and entering mysticism'.

Further down the list there are the more predictable pauses that come between sounds. These may be the moments of only relative silence (usually broken by coughing!) between the movements in a piece of music, between sentences when a compulsive talker stops to take breath ('That man's silence', said the character Mr Spinks in Thomas Hardy's *Under the Greenwood Tree*, talking about a garrulous acquaintance, 'is wonderful to listen to') or on a usually busy main road when there is a pause in the traffic flow or even in bed when the snorer who may be lying beside you chooses laboriously to turn over and to breathe quietly for a while (before, inevitably, starting again to snore). Then there can be pauses unsought and mechanical in origin. These are the ones that come, for example, when there is a power cut or when the battery of your walkman runs out, or when the mobile telephone you are using unexpectedly goes dead.

For the hearing impaired, however, there are obviously thousands of pauses every day, which can only be disconcerting. These occur when you have not heard clearly, or haven't heard at all, what your best friend or whoever may be saying to you. It may be a lengthy bit of communication or a brief comment of only passing interest. Perhaps, if you were not watching his or her face, and especially the lips, you missed the inflexion as he or she raised their voice with a question. For many of us this can be socially very unsettling and conspicuously so when you miss the key words in a friend's anecdote and you are uncomfortably aware that everyone else is falling about laughing. It can also be desperately frustrating to miss out on a word or two of intense seriousness.

For those who wear hearing aids there are also the pauses, long as well as short, which may be mechanically induced. But they are no less unsettling. The battery in your hearing aid may indeed suddenly fail or the aid itself may be defective or it may not be working. A friend dropped his in the bathroom sink one morning, just as he was about to shave, with the result that he had several days of often distressing silence he had not bargained for while it was being repaired. An attack of catarrh can block – with or without a hearing aid – the detail of the sounds that you are normally able to distinguish.

Sounds can be individual, simultaneous or concerted. Sounds, like silences, can be welcome, even soothing, like agreeable music or good conversation, but they can be harsh and unwelcome, like the scraping of a metal saucepan with a metal spoon. There is a medical condition called recruitment, which is about the unwished-for impingement of apparently exaggerated sounds. It is a moot point whether these should include, for instance, the sound of the otherwise delightful small child who wakes and wants attention at the very moment when sleep is an infinitely preferable option!

There are many sounds you miss, in every sense of the word, when you lose your hearing but also many that you seem to gain. Some are more obvious than others. Everybody who loses some hearing will sooner or later make a reference to bird-song or to the sound of even the most gentle breeze in the trees that are no longer available. Perhaps, having lost your hearing, you sigh heavily but you are able to accept that sort of thing as a new fact of life – although there is no reason why you should accept it – however, you may sigh less heavily at not being able to make confident use of a mobile phone.

Some losses are odd. It can be disconcerting, as I have said, not to hear tap water running, and it can be bizarre not to hear yourself turning the pages of the book you are reading. Equally disconcerting, on the other hand, can be the sounds that you find yourself starting to pick out once you have a hearing aid in your ear. The central heating may be noisier – even though it's only a hum – than you bargained for, an electric kettle on the boil can kill even the most casual conversation stone dead, while the tick of an electric clock may intrude and even the electric toaster may start emitting mysterious sounds that you never even suspected existed. In the sleepless early hours it can be difficult to differentiate between what sounds like soft footfalls on the stair: is the semi-detached neighbour setting off for his early-morning shift, is it your partner creeping downstairs for a glass of water or is it merely your own heart doing its rhythmic duty and apparently thumping against your ribs because of the unusual position in which you are lying in bed?

Sounds, unless they are cacophonic, are not the same thing as noise. Noise, after all, is a matter for argument, even (if you live near an offending airport or have a recalcitrant neighbour) for public controversy. Books will go on being written about noise, parliamentarians will go on legislating against it, on the assumption that too much of it is by no means a good thing, and statisticians will find new ways of announcing that far too many of the population of Britain are exposed to unacceptably high levels of it. Even so, despite the continued warnings of the damage that can result, especially in the form of unwanted stress or hearing loss, its effects for the majority will go on being ignored. At the same time, of course, there is also noise which is ostensibly pleasurable, as in the case of a party, an animated discussion or interest group (even an anti-noise group) or the new shopping centre, the theatre before the curtain goes up or the cinema.

Invariably, the downside is when you are unable to control what you hear and your privacy is invaded. Silences as well as sounds can be invaders. Jack Ashley has recorded that when he went deaf it was like 'drowning in a sea of silence'. I have known several individuals who have defined their hearing loss as a sort of underwater way of living. Richard Parker, a friend of mine and a family man who lives in a North Yorkshire village, was used to quietness before he lost his hearing, but he still recalls the new silence, which accompanied his overnight loss of hearing, several years ago, as 'very, very frightening'.

A corollary to the experience of Richard Parker is the experience of one Kate Holiday, a tinnitus sufferer, who wrote in a recent issue of *Hearing Therapy* magazine about her life, living in France, with tinnitus – a condition which apparently came to her after the breakdown of her marriage. 'Like most people in my position,' she wrote, 'I think I only began to treasure utter silence when it was lost . . . My tolerance of tinnitus does improve, [but] still, sometimes up a mountain, I do miss the sound of silence.'

FOUR

Resources and remedies

I T IS CALLED presbycusis, and it is, according to those who know, the natural hearing loss that you may expect to experience as you get older. It is emphatically not a disease (says the textbook), but more than half of all people over sixty are affected by it. The cause is a deterioration in the inner ear, the cochlea, and the tiny blood vessels it contains, coupled with the loss of the very small hair cells there that monitor sounds on their way to the brain. There was a flurry of excitement in the middle of 2003 when it was announced there had been a breakthrough in a science laboratory in the USA where, it was said, a way had been found of replacing these cells in very small animals. British research is being conducted in the same area using newts, and here, too, excitement could soon be in the air. These are welcome straws in the wind and not the first in this particular area, but it was also indicative that there is still a long way to go.

For the time being the loss of these cells usually becomes apparent to the man or woman in the street (and men are more susceptible than women) when they have passed fifty and when other people become more difficult to understand and seem, to the hearer, to have unaccountably started mumbling when they speak. At the same time, crowded places that have been routinely visited for a good time or for some social relaxation are suddenly transformed into places that are claustrophobic and intolerably noisy. Then you may realize you are not hearing the front door bell as well as you used to or that the telephone's ring does not seem as loud as it was. But, finally, there comes a moment when it dawns on you, or it is made clear by someone who is close to you and tactful by nature, that you are finding it surprisingly hard work to keep up with conversation in a group. That dawning can be a very disconcerting, even distressing, moment.

And now comes the crunch. You begin to realize that people have to repeat themselves – sometimes more than once – when they are talking to you. However much you try to treat this complication with a sort of nonchalance, shrugging it off initially, you soon begin to ask yourself what on earth is really going on. Defeat (which is what it feels like) comes when after some final, and futile, attempts at prevarication you reach a point where you feel you just want to run, to get away from the black hole that seems to be opening up in front of you. But there is no escape.

It is usually the high-frequency sounds, and especially the higher-pitched consonants, which are the first to become distorted and go beyond reach. This is why it is the voices of women and children that are the first to go missing. One consequence of this among many is that it can mean the plural can become indistinguishable from singular. As the RNID cheerily points out, you reach a point where you have to beware, if you are in this vulnerable state, of someone seeming to offer – or to want to accept – what sounds like 'a big kiss' when the offering is only of a biscuit. Mishearings can lead to tragedy and tension, but they can also be fun, of sorts, despite the hidden potential for being calamitous. Denis Healey, once a distinguished Labour Cabinet Minister, acknowledged that in his late seventies he would get into the habit of leaning forward in front of his television set, hoping for interesting personal revelations, every time he heard the words Stena Sealink (the name of a shipping line). He was under the impression, he said, that someone somewhere was, once again, taking his name in vain.

In fact, of course, the damage to the hair cells in the cochlea comes, in older people like myself, from what is gently called natural wear and tear. But the same sort of damage can come to all sorts of people by a number of other routes. There may be an inheritance factor or, in rarer instances, there may be what the research charity Defeating Deafness calls a diet-and-lifestyle factor. Obviously, serious head injuries can cause major hearing problems, as can working for long periods in excessively noisy environments. A baby's ears can be damaged if the mother has German measles (rubella) during early pregnancy and also during the process of birth itself. In addition, there are some drugs which are capable of doing harm, including certain antibiotics, diuretics and even aspirin. Perforated ear drums can occasionally be repaired or even heal by themselves, but problems arise if they are caused by sudden loud noises such as fireworks, bombs or even a car back-firing. Prolonged spells of swimming under water, including diving, can be dangerous. So can the old-wives' recommendation of using pre-heated olive oil in the ear – if the oil is too hot.

In the first instance, it has to be the family doctor who is meant to refer you and your problem to the nearest audiologist, a person who is usually hospital based. But GPs vary, and even the best-intentioned of them may have to be persuaded. There are plenty of instances on record where the GP has said to one of his or her older patients that they should go away and think of something else. 'Of course your hearing may be failing,' says the tetchy doctor, 'but what can you expect when you're getting older?' It is heartening to know that pressures for deaf and hearing-impaired people have actively been trying hard to change doctors' attitudes, even to the extent of producing a printed guide to help them to communicate more effectively.

But just how penetrable is your average GP? One of the bullet points in the guide is that it is helpful to the patient if the doctor actually looks at them when he or she is talking and takes the minimal trouble to pause for a moment in what he or she may be writing or reading on a piece of paper. (One hearing professional I read about has described how he arranged to address a doctors' surgery on how they should deal with patients with hearing loss. On the appointed day, the reception and nursing staff attended diligently but no doctors!)

Perceived hostility in the GP's surgery is something that some hard-of-hearing patients have grown used to, and there have been surveys in recent years which have sought to quantify the costs of this hostility, to both the patient and to the NHS. I give some details of this research in a later chapter. But not all GPs are intractable and apparently unwilling to listen – some may even have hearing problems of their own. It is always possible that your GP may be one of those, even in these straitened times, who is up to the minute. He or she may have some basic electronic testing equipment and the knowledge to ask what sounds you can and cannot hear satisfactorily. Some doctors may work to a different level of satisfaction, through the clever use of voice and whisper tests (when the voice in conversation suddenly changes to a whisper to test reaction) or through the skilful use of a tuning fork. There are several revealing tests that can be carried out with the fork, which for centuries has been a tried and tested instrument, but it still takes skill – and a delicate touch – on the right bone area to use one.

The GP is only the first step. The next is getting an appointment to see a qualified audiologist, who specializes in hearing and balance and related matters, or an ear, nose and throat specialist. This is not an easy task, and access, as in so many health matters, may depend on availability of such people, which in turn depends on your postcode. The average waiting time to see a hearing specialist, according to the government's own figures (published at the end of 2003), is longer than for almost any other.

One of the troubles with audiologists is that they vary not only in availability but also in competence. For one thing, they are a relatively new phenomenon: the word audiology, which covers a range of different specialisms, was only used for the first time in very recent years. But change is in the air, and after too long a period of what might be called a process of groping in the foothills as a Cinderella calling, it is gaining in eminence and indisputably strengthening its position as a nationally recognized profession. Like many professions (real or aspiring) it has already found time to spawn its own hierarchies. This means that despite obvious overlaps in capabilities an audiological scientist is not necessarily the same person as an audiologist, who is not the same as a hearing therapist and certainly not the same as a mere hearing-aid dispenser. I have read of a hearing-aid technician who, on being asked a fairly elementary question by his patient about the nature of his hearing problem, told him, 'Sorry, I can't help you there. You'll have to go back to your doctor.'

After a protracted debate the practitioners have finally agreed that all audiologists should be educated at least to degree level and that the new graduates who emerge from this (government-supported) dispensation will be going into practice towards the end of 2006. A national register will monitor the qualifications and up-to-dateness of all practitioners. Even so, the specialists are agreed, modernization of the service – which involves testing babies only a few hours after birth as well as everyone else in need – will take many years to complete.

All sorts of factors and preconditions are associated with hearing loss. One of these is known as vestibular imbalance. This is what you and I would recognize as a particular form of dizziness, caused in part by the ear passing faulty sounds or signals, perhaps through faulty canals inside the ear, to an unreceptive or confused brain. Such imbalance may precede or accompany hearing loss, but specialists say there is usually no cause–effect relationship. Similar symptoms, after all, may also be brought on through the use of unfamiliar drugs or through poor circulation of the blood and even, rarely, in the first phase of wearing a new pair of glasses.

Ménière's disease is one which can affect one ear (initially) and can also lead to a seriously impaired sense of balance, with the sufferer routinely walking into door jambs instead of through the doorway. One of my lip-reading friends often has black bruises all over one or both of his hands caused by just this affliction. Such dizzy spells can last several hours at a time. Happily the friend does not obviously display any of the associated side-effects, which include loss of confidence and anxiety and even depression. But then the warm and friendly (and therapeutic) environment of the lip-reading class itself may well be an effective antidote. At the same time there are some sedative drugs that can be taken to combat the dizziness, and the person concerned is advised to lay off alcohol, tobacco, salt and coffee. (Now I know why he always has orange juice during the class coffee break!)

Middle-ear disease and glue ear, which affects four out of five children under five, can occasionally bring on dizziness and sickness as well as hearing loss. Short-term alleviation can be achieved through pills, suppositories and, in most severe cases, through surgery, but all these conditions are among those which can precipitate short- or longer-term hearing loss. Otosclerosis, caused by what is known as bone overgrowth and more commonly affecting women than men, may be hereditary but is something which can be operated on – but this remains a controversial area of debate.

Ageing, and the deterioration of physical/mechanical equipment that accompanies it, remain the commonest cause of hearing loss. Apart from Ménière's disease, there can also be hidden dangers in contracting meningitis or mumps or measles, where some hearing loss may ensue.

On the other hand, away from the sickbed there can also be hidden dangers in living or working or even enjoying yourself in an unusually noisy environment. Thus, the front line of battle, where bombs may be exploding, or the unprotected factory production line, where the machinery may be noisy, or the work of portering all day at a noisy railway station, or even the pleasure of playing as a member of a pop group or a symphony orchestra can be seriously problematic. At the same time there is the statistic that one child in five hundred is born with significantly impaired hearing and often to normally hearing parents.

Once the individual disoriented by hearing loss or deafness and the trained specialist, whether NHS or private, confront each other, the search starts in earnest for an appropriate treatment. However, as the waiting list suggests, the said confrontation can be difficult to facilitate. Although the number of deaf and hearing-impaired people is continuing to grow, the number of qualified audiologists who are able to treat them with real competence is certainly not. If you are just about to join the queue, which could, statistically be several thousand people long (if all those who could benefit joined it), be patient and try not to be exasperated by the waiting. But if, in fact, you are driven into a decision to go private, then it is essential that you should check with an otologist or with the Hearing Aid Council that the dispenser you are using is approved and registered.

The Hearing Aid Council, which is based in Milton Keynes and deals specifically with complaints about suppliers of hearing aids, is an organization with teeth. It currently handles around two hundred complaints a year – representing a slight fall over preceding years – and, according to its latest report, called twenty-three hearing-aid dispensers and five companies before its disciplinary committee to face a total of 164 different charges. Almost every charge was found proved and appropriate fines imposed. One company, known as Ambassador Hearing Healthcare (previously known as Harley Hearing Aid Centres), was scrutinized for nearly two weeks by the Council's disciplinary committee before being struck off the Council's register and its directors heavily fined.

But, whether you go NHS or private, what you are usually after in the first instance is a hearing aid. This is a device for which the first patent was granted at the very end of the nineteenth century and which reached a significant landmark, making use of electronic possibilities, half a century later. For a long time it was a cumbersome object with unsightly attachments; today it is smaller and more streamlined, unobtrusive even, something to put in your ear which amplifies sounds with an attachment that loops around behind your ear and transmits what you want to hear.

But once you find yourself in the presence of your chosen specialist there are snags before they can even start to treat you. The exchanges between you may be built on totally different perceptions. Yours is that of the patient concerned, almost certainly trying, perhaps with great difficulty, to come to terms with a confusing, perplexing and deeply personal problem. Something has happened that will probably change your life – for ever. Your specialist, on the other hand, is simply doing his or her job.

While a new quality of hearing, however it is to be achieved, is clearly a priority, a whole range of accompanying concerns, some of them extremely difficult to put into words, also have to be addressed. The specialists in their white coats may be very deft at examining the inside of your ear, but they know very well, as the textbooks constantly reiterate, that their otoscopes and other instruments are not adequate for dealing with the social and psychological complications thrown up by hearing loss. Besides, the queue in the corridor outside is getting longer. The result is that today's health-care professionals, as I read in an American magazine in early 2004, are besieged by managed, health-care-driven 'hurried appointments' and are pressured to get the job done as quickly as possible.

Even where rudimentary help is at hand there is a lack of clear mutual understanding before treatment to choose an appropriate hearing aid can begin. You are installed in a soundproof little booth, wired up to a machine with mysteriously flickering dials and you have massive headphones placed over your ears. You are shown something soft which you have to press when you hear the tones that are being relayed to you. The results of your different responses are reproduced in graphic form on a graph called an audiogram and the extent to which your ears, at this moment in time, are actually taking in or distorting sounds can be determined. Your hearing loss is calibrated, procedures decided and your future way of life circumscribed in a totally new way in less than half an hour.

The first question arises before even the first tone has been tried. It lies in the very fact that hearing tests too often concentrate on measuring the patient's ability to hear what are scientifically determined pure tones, bleeps which are electronically produced and electronically measured. If that seems OK by you and you think it's a good start, pause for a moment. For this is not reality. Most of the sounds that we encounter in real life, hearing or not hearing, are anything but pure or scientifically determined. They come at us in all sorts of contexts, from varying distances, in different tones and at different frequencies. Everybody, in other words, has different vocal cords, and everybody speaks differently. 'Speech audiometry', when the patient has to register hearing actual words, is clearly an under-utilized resource.

Once the level of loss for each ear has been determined, by plotting the results on the audiogram, you will be presented a few weeks later with an appropriate hearing aid. Usually it consists of the plastic blob to go in your ear and the mechanics in a curved little box behind it. But they come in different guises. There is also the body-worn aid, housed in a small box you can carry in a pocket or attach to your lapel. There are bone-conduction or bone-anchored aids which may be effective but which lack sophistication whichever way you look at them. Another aid can be attached to your spectacle frame, but it cannot be separated and presents problems if the specs or the aid needs replacing or repairing. Acceptance of the hearing aid, in whatever form, can be a hugely complicated moment, one that can be met with relief, with fear, with joy or even with a sort of residual disbelief that the thing, and the compulsory wearing of it, is really necessary after all.

Attitudes have changed. In *Handbook of Hearing Aids*, published in New York in 1940, there was an acknowledgement that in the 1920s 'electrical aids for hearing were a horror to the deafened who wore them and to those that did not wear them'. The former felt that any such device was 'too conspicuous', while the latter, on giving any instrument an 'unfair' trial, heard 'a jumble of promiscuous noises', because of the carbon particles that jumped around haphazardly inside the ear. At that time, of course, the hearing aid was still not in general use. Reading the book, said a guest writer in the foreword, would make the deafened person more unselfconscious and make him feel it is 'more than worth his while' to wear an instrument that will allow him to relax and hear conversation without effort.

In most of these cases, by way of preparation for a modern hearing aid, a plastic mould will have been made at the same time as your hearing test to fit the sculptural peculiarities of your own ear. Once you have put the thing in place – and it may take a bit of pride-swallowing to wear it for the first time, not to mention the physical discomfort – you will find that it distorts at the same time as it enhances what you are able to hear. But the very fact that you are once again actually able to hear at all can be enough – as a seasoned deafness coordinator told me – to make you smile inside, and, when someone starts talking (audibly!), that can be enough to bring back a neglected feeling of some delight.

There are several different sorts even of the most common type of hearing aid. It is a device that is continually undergoing development. This, in turn, suggests that if you are not using the NHS you should beware of what may seem to be over-spending on your first one, for the simple reason that it could be superseded within a year, or even a month, of purchase. The most usual type, known in the trade as BTE, is worn behind the ear. Another fills the external cavity of the ear and is known as ITE (in the ear) or, if it sits in the ear canal, as ITC or CIC (in the canal or completely in the canal).

One of the first aids designed to amplify sound through the use of electric power was used by Queen Alexandra at the coronation of her husband King Edward VII in 1902, in which she was an active participant. How much she heard and how good the quality of the sound was has not been recorded, but the device was mains-powered and it was deemed – understandably – to be too unwieldy to be developed for more general or commercial use. Pictures of the period show hand-held devices that look more like machine guns than hearing aids.

It has been estimated that most of the people using hearing aids – nearly 2 million – are making do with what British researchers have decided recently are 'unusable and poor quality' analogue devices based on technology that is between twenty and thirty years old. For many users, by no means all, they seem to work to varying degrees of satisfaction. A friend of mine was thrilled when he got his first NHS hearing aid and put on a recording of what he thought was a familiar piece of piano music. There were all sorts of nuances which suddenly came to him, he said, that he had not heard before. Another friend, suffering with acquired and profound deafness, has had to live with the fact that in their case there would be little or no benefit from using an ordinary hearing aid. A third, much younger, friend was told to try lip-reading, although with a quiet reminder that if lip-reading ever came to be regarded as a language, and if they went on to university education, then students using it while at their place of study could be charged fees for the extra teaching responsibilities involved.

For many, that new-found contentment may be enough. For others – an unknown number – the hearing aid is an embarrassing excrescence which is simply too visible and which draws attention to their disability. For some wearers they are too intricate or too technical and the tiny controls, for the microphone, the amplifier and the earphone itself, are barely manageable. If you have arthritis in your fingers the required bit of fiddling may be too much and the temptation may be to stick the thing away in a drawer. Then, if your hearing deteriorates further or if your ear changes shape, which it does, you may have to think again. But it is a common complaint among wearers that, apart from the too few hearing therapists offering their services, there is little or no help, let alone after-sales service, on how to make best use of them. Some sociological or similar research into the wearer's relationship with his or her hearing aid would surely yield some fascinating results.

In my own experience I soon found that I had to be prepared for what I can only call a darkish-brown overlay of sound to the unexpectedly deep tone of the person who is talking to me. I also had to get used to the unexpected intrusion of sounds I was never previously aware of. Hence, where before it was always predictably difficult to hear what individual people were saying in a crowded room, it had now become almost impossible. Like many thousands of others, I have stopped going to parties, reunions and other gatherings which had previously been such an important part of life. Some individuals with hearing loss speak extra-loudly, which means that even deaf clubs, where two or three such people may be in the same room, can be very noisy places! The distortion from loudspeakers is also magnified to unmanageable levels. Where the public address system at the railway station was previously simply unclear, it had now become a cacophonous parody of its former self. It goes without saying that for some people with hearing loss travel by train can be a very stressful experience.

Since the preceding paragraph was first written I have learned that some audiologists and hearing therapists advise that newly acquired hearing aids should only be worn for short spells – perhaps thirty minutes at a time – in the first few days in order for the wearer to became accustomed to their capabilities. This sounds very acceptable advice and should surely be given by all those who are involved in dispensing such aids. It cannot be over-emphasized that the taking of the aid and the decision to wear it, or not, are often enormous to the person concerned. A retired professor I know told me he was scared to go to the hospital to collect his, and others have spoken of breaking down in tears at the prospect. In Germany, I have read, it takes hearing-impaired people an *average of thirteen years* to consult the relevant specialist.

Digital aids are the ones to watch. As I write, government ministers are promising that digital hearing aids, providing modern technology through the use of a very small computer chip which has been honed to meet individual requirements, will soon be available, free of charge, to all who need them. But with all the sophistication in the world, even digitalized hearing aids, says the relevant literature, cannot restore perfect hearing in the way that a new pair of glasses can restore sight. The best-quality aids, it is conceded, will not necessarily make everything clear – 'a badly fitted digital', I have read, 'is not better than a badly fitted analogue' – and if your knowledge of basic technology happens to be limited you may find them difficult to handle. (In August 2004 the RNID was able to report that 280,000 people had been fitted with digital hearing aids on the NHS – a small victory for relentless campaigning. But, with millions waiting in the wings for similar equipment, there is still a long way to go.)

If it's any consolation, just remember that you are not alone, not by any means, if you have acquired a hearing aid and, for whatever reason, you have declined to use it. Nor are you by any means alone if you suddenly feel cast adrift, in need of advice and support. That blob of moulded plastic in your ear is not a life raft. The need for counsellors, or even trained therapists in this area, has hardly been explored. Of one thing you can be almost certain: if you take your worries back to the clinic which supplied your aid it will be a different audiologist who is on duty.

Until recently a very important, and not uncontroversial, development had been in the use being made of cochlear implants – used where the inner-ear hair cells have been irreparably (at this moment in time) damaged and where the person concerned is severely or profoundly deaf. Once again there is a microphone that transmits sounds to a processing device, which is itself connected by tiny wires to a transmitter inside the ear. A total of some 50,000 people are now said to be using cochlear implants, but it is still the case that not everyone approves of their use – on the grounds that it is interfering with nature – particularly with very small children. Meanwhile some exciting research is said to be going on at British universities into their potential.

The letter columns of the specialist journals aimed at people with hearing loss are routinely filled with cries of desperation and dismay from individuals, with and without hearing aids, who find themselves overwhelmed by their new-found sense of isolation and, in many cases, loneliness. Depression, it is known, is something which comes as a matter of course to many who suffer hearing loss; those who are born deaf tend not to suffer in the same way. Withdrawal is also not uncommon. Close relationships, inevitably, suffer – sometimes irreparably. *De facto* separation and divorce proceedings, if not *de jure*, are known to climb in households where there is hearing loss: one recent survey has shown that 40 per cent of respondents say communication with their partner has become 'more difficult'. Tension and stress as a result of mishearings and/or misunderstandings certainly become routine.

The responsible editors of the journals to whom the sufferers write do their best. They regularly spell out their sympathy with such people, but the RNID, for one, also adopts a no-nonsense, tell-it-like-it-is approach to the problem. You may find, it says, that you need to learn some new personal skills, and you sometimes have to assert yourself . . . But remember, it adds rather disingenuously, there is always help available. Ah, but, you may reply, is it available and is it really viable for the harassed individual having a first-class row with his or her partner or for the poor pensioner, living alone, at three in the morning when that person cannot sleep because he or she is being driven to distraction by the strange sounds or the unfamiliar quietness that now assail? And what of the deaf person who is three or four times as likely as his or her hearing neighbour to be unemployed, or the hard-of-hearing person who is grossly underpaid or who is capable of more than the semi-skilled or unskilled work he or she is obliged to do?

Not everyone with hearing loss fits into the socially well-adjusted mould, and not everyone is assertive or even gregarious enough to rush out to join a local support group or lip-reading class. It is almost universal among deaf people, wrote an American columnist called Henry Kisor a dozen or so years ago, that they want to cause hearing people as little fuss as possible and that as a result they finish up in a role that is 'self-effacing and diffident to the point of invisibility'. But then there is the specialist's view that young people are inclined to exaggerate their disability, while older people play theirs down. Lip-reading, anyway, is something some people have an aptitude for (as with languages), and it is a stressful pursuit if you are not in the mood.

In other words, deaf and hard-of-hearing people cannot turn into social animals overnight if it is not in their nature to do so, even when it may be for their own good. If they live in a small community where every act may be talked about they may not want to let their problems be exposed. At the end of the day, they may not be able to articulate their feelings, and they may feel that sense of stigma. 'You may have to assert yourself sometimes,' says Auntie RNID, smacking you tetchily on the wrist, 'by reminding people to face you and speak clearly ... and in a good light.' On the other hand, when social contact has become an effort, it just may not be as easy as that.

Tinnitus, which varies in degree from a gentle internal buzzing or whistling to even a shrieking or roaring that nobody else can hear, is something else that comes to many people, especially when they are older. As many as one in four of the population are thought to suffer, and for nearly 4 million people it is a permanent problem, more prevalent in people who have passed middle age and also have hearing loss. It, too, can come as a result of being subjected to loud noise, after illness or as a result of head injuries and also, in the more susceptible, to individuals who have suffered some emotional upset or, occasionally, who have been taking drugs. There are compact discs available which are intended to soothe and relax their buyers with tinnitus: they offer 'tranquil music [which] helps you to drift away from your everyday problems'. The problems don't go away, of course, but . . .

A couple of conditions often associated with both tinnitus and presbycusis are called hyperacusis and recruitment. Hyperacusis is where everyday noises, ordinarily acceptable, suddenly become unbearable and where following a conversation, if there are more than two or three people in the room, can be very difficult. If you are at home you will find that dishes seem unaccountably to be clattering on to the table, loudspeaker announcements or vehicles in the street, especially emergency-service vehicles with sirens, seem almost life-threatening, while the average vacuum cleaner seems to be a monster that is engulfing the whole house with its noise, and so on.

Loudness recruitment is an inner-ear condition where weak sounds may not be heard but where louder sounds, such as those just listed, can cause pain that may, in some cases, lead to panic attacks. As with hearing loss, there is no definitive cure for either of these conditions, but both are treatable, up to a point, and some alleviation is possible.

FIVE
'Cures' and detours

Any attempt to trace the ways in which deafness and hearing loss and other aural problems have been dealt with over the centuries can be confusing as well as rewarding and is sometimes disturbingly entertaining. Many of the routes taken have led up blind alleys and, while there have been many well-meaning and deeply compassionate practitioners and theorists, their basic assumptions were on occasion highly questionable. The otologist, as an individual with sophisticated training who specializes in problems associated with the ear, is, as I have noted, even in the twenty-first century, a relatively new creature and one who does not always agree with his or her colleagues on courses of treatment proposed. This is for the simple reason that otologists' approaches, even those which are based on the best of intentions, can start from markedly differing standpoints depending on their own special interests or expertise. Add to this the fact that at many NHS clinics the audiologist or whoever is on duty may well vary from one appointment to the next, and the hapless hard-of-hearing person, waiting in yet another dismal queue, may well emit a heavy sigh. The NHS, I read shortly after a routine visit to the clinic, needs more than money to achieve its most worthwhile objectives; it also needs more efficiency, more flexibility and a more humane approach in the interpretation of its rules. And that is a view I have heard many times.

Some basic questions have to be unravelled before lines of historical thinking can be described. In tracing the methods that, through time, have been intended to support and treat individuals who may be deaf or who have hearing loss, and attitudes to their condition, there are many distractions and false starts. We have moved on, for instance, from the thinking of the seventeenth-century herbalist Nicholas Culpeper, who recommended that the leaves and stalks of the sow thistle should be boiled in the oil of bitter almonds and wrapped in the peel of a pomegranate as 'a sure remedy for deafness, singings, etc.' And mistletoe tea, as a treatment for nerve deafness, has little popular credence nowadays. In other words, the territory, whether one wishes it or not, is one of many disciplines, proven and unproven. This is the area not just of ear, nose and throat pathology but also of philosophy, linguistics, sociology and psychology, as well as multifarious and esoteric branches of medicine. But it is also the somewhat murky area where superstition and fears of the unknown have also played their part. So long as there have been gullible patients, there have been suspect remedies and cures. In preparing these pages I have scoured the medical shelves of many diverse bookshops but, outside the specialist sections, have found little of comfort. Looking through the index at the back of what might appear to be a promising tome, taken at random off the shelf, and searching for references to the deaf or to deafness, you find nothing, but you do find that alphabetically you are disconcertingly close to plenty of references to death. And when you switch your search to hearing, again you may find nothing, although heart attack, heart failure and heart trouble are all near by.

There has always been a great deal of mystery and incomprehension about deafness and hearing loss. When people are born unable to hear or speak they are more or less alone. But what are they thinking and what is *their* attitude to the world they perceive around them? How does, how should, the world begin to relate to them? It takes little imagination to understand the reservations and feelings of suspicion that could arise between two different sorts of people – the hearing and the not-hearing – who have no ready means of communicating with each other. If the only sounds an individual can make are different sorts of roar, to express anger or impatience with people's attitudes or possibly amusement and enthusiasm – only part of the difficulties of day-to-day living – it is hardly surprising that wariness and/or hostility enter the equation. Hardly surprising either that the individual concerned can finish up being ostracized, living alone with his or her wretchedly incomprehensible disability.

Between 3000 and 4000 years ago the Ancient Egyptians seemed to have a relatively humane approach. Some modern historians have suggested that they may well have been compassionate towards people with hearing loss, largely because they were also known to have a measure of respect for people who had little or no sight. Such people were taught music and other arts, such as the art of massage, and some became distinguished as poets and musicians and were encouraged to find a role through participation in religious services.

The Ancient Greeks, who were in time to invade Egypt, had, as I have already noted, their own ways of assimilating local ideas and customs. But as far as deafness was concerned, the allegedly civilized Greeks seem to have had more in common with the Nazis of twentieth-century Germany than the Egyptians. In the seventh century BC it was customary for the congenitally disabled, including those who apparently had no hearing, to be destroyed as soon as possible after birth. The authorities' view was that such creatures should not be a burden on society. The exterminators who collaborated with Hitler, one suspects, would have understood; the least they wanted for the deaf was that they should be sterilized. Despite their social sophistication and the relics that remain of the trumpeted glories of Greece, the society was one that was decidedly conservative and sometimes downright brutal, and certainly unimaginative, in many sensitive policy areas.

Hippocrates, born on the Greek island of Kos in the fifth century BC, was one of the most accomplished medical men in antiquity, a figure still regarded with some veneration. This father of medicine and his several followers made great play of the links they claimed to find between congenital or pre-lingual deafness and speechlessness, and many theories were advanced in their time for the causes and possible cures of one or both conditions. Among the causes they suggested were apoplexy or some form of brain damage. At the same time, however, they believed that individuals who were born deaf were incapable of learning to speak. At least someone was giving the matter serious thought, and theories, even if they were erroneous, were giving rise to argument, and this must be counted more acceptable than unimaginative indifference.

The oddball Greek philosopher Socrates was one whose views in many areas went against the grain of popular thought. Although among the dwindling band of classical scholars who are today still revered for their wisdom, he was in fact condemned to death in his own time – more than

2400 years ago – for corrupting the young and promoting the interests of unacceptable gods. He wrote nothing himself, but his views and opinions were noted by his equally distinguished follower Plato who regurgitated them for posterity. It is through Plato that we know that Socrates was one of the first people to speak with some sympathy of the special difficulties encountered by individuals who were deaf. Thought, he argued, rather than words, was the conversation of the soul, and if we had no voice and no ability to speak, and yet we wished to communicate, would we not do as people that are mute already do, namely, signify our meanings through the use of our hands, our head and other parts of the body?

Here, if you like, was a scratchy acknowledgement of the potential, and perhaps also the efficacy, of rudimentary sign language. A very small child cries and gesticulates – that is, signs – wildly when it is hungry. When it is a little older and preoccupied or tired or not feeling too good, it signs again, perhaps by glumly sucking its thumb. When affection is called for or is on offer, then smiles or even kisses may be offered or exchanged. This is sign language at its most elementary. It is basic communication, and it has always been with us, from almost the beginning of our lives.

But ever since Socrates sign language, used in various forms by deaf people among themselves as a *de facto* language, has had, and still has, a rough ride. In what turned out to be its most cathartic year, at the International Conference of the Deaf in Milan in 1880, it was to suffer outright rejection from those who demanded, seemingly without equivocation, that deaf people should be taught, somehow or other, to speak. This was presumably on the basic assumption that the deaf and the hard of hearing would be able to grasp the significance and the need for such things as words, however clumsily articulated, even though they could not grasp these same words through their own ears. British Sign Language has only very recently been recognized as a language in its own right, but in the summer of 2003 a march through London by several thousand deaf people, culminating in a Trafalgar Square rally, called for more 'protection' for BSL and for more legal rights for users.

Aristotle, another Greek philosopher, was born fifteen years after Socrates' execution and managed, in his own way, to carry on the business of philosophical thinking. He had been a pupil himself of Socrates' note-taker Plato, and he was more rigorously disciplined in his thinking than the ruminative Socrates, advancing several theories of his own on the nature and behaviour of animals, including human animals. Although Aristotle's theories were not always as charitable towards disadvantaged animals as were those of Socrates, nevertheless Charles Darwin, writing two thousand years later, was constrained to acknowledge his own debt to the seminal thinking of Aristotle in his writings on evolution.

Aristotle evidently had a ruthless streak, and it is to the credit of many of Darwin's predecessors who thought about and actively sought to treat different levels of hearing loss and deafness over the preceding five hundred or so years that they sought in many cases, but not all, to bypass the thinking of Aristotle. It is now generally agreed that Aristotle's declaration that the human being's capacity for hearing – that is, hearing ideas – constituted 'the greatest contribution to intelligence' and his converse views about not hearing were therefore directly and indirectly responsible for holding back education, and remedial help, for the hearing impaired for fifteen hundred years. Aristotle would tolerate no half-measures in his determination to encourage the development of what he would define as a perfect society.

Language, according to Aristotle, was a prerequisite for thought, as well as a means of articulating it. He reasoned that since the deaf could not hear, they would not learn to talk. Since they could not talk properly, they would not be able to think constructively and formulate ideas. These were individuals, in the philosopher's view, who quite simply lacked the vital and life-enhancing commodity called reason, which meant they also lacked essential understanding. Since deafness was, by his extrapolation, an untreatable imperfection it should not be encouraged. The deaf were retarded, and that was that: total rejection.

The Romans, like the followers of Aristotle, had their own superstitions. The father in the early Roman family set-up was someone who inherited some patriarchal customs from the Greeks. He would routinely arrogate to himself the powers of judge and jury in his own household, and the family would not question the general rule that new-born children with physical disabilities, including deafness, should be flung to drown as speedily as possible in the nearest available fast-flowing water. This demonstrable lack of compassion made compromise difficult, but more enlightened policy-makers seem to have showed themselves instinctively more capable of granting more basic human rights.

More progressive law-makers took steps to promote the view that the disabled should in fact be offered some sort of training, in spite of their disabilities. They did so despite the fact that the ordinary Roman stuck doggedly to the Aristotelian view, that deaf people were simply not capable of being educated and were therefore expendable At some point, however, this view was overturned from the centre, and there are records of the emergence of successful deaf farmers, tradespeople and even front-line soldiers. One deaf man, Quintus Pedius, son of a Roman consul, was encouraged to become an eminent painter, although he died young.

By the sixth century AD, when Justinian became Emperor of Byzantium, the tide had turned completely. In the year 529 he embarked on the codification of Roman Law, a move through which he was to have a significant effect on later law-makers throughout Europe. In provisions for the disabled he sought to differentiate between the congenitally affected and those who became disabled in later life. Those who were born deaf and dumb, he said, should not be allowed to make a bequest or a will; on the other hand, those who lost their hearing or became dumb as a result of disease, or who became 'tongue-tied' in the course of their lives, should face no such restrictions.

The first Christians, meanwhile, were emboldened by propositions that they assumed came from God, as revealed in the Bible. This meant they had their own ways of explaining deafness, of dealing with it, and even, by way of miracles, curing it. God, as it is told in the Old Testament, orders a hesitant Moses to pull himself together when the old man announces that he is reluctant, because he might be tongue-tied in explaining his leadership principles, to set about liberating the Jews from Egypt. God will have none of this: 'It is I who makes a man dumb or deaf. I will help your speech . . .' Problem apparently solved.

Jesus was to be somewhat less peremptory. He had his own rather rudimentary ways of dealing with a man presented to him who was deaf and had speech impediments. According to the New Testament account given by the evangelist Mark, he took the man so afflicted to one side, away from the crowd, and did a number of things no self-respecting audiologist would surely ever do. He put his fingers in the man's ears, spat and then touched the man's tongue. Then, perhaps rather as an audiologist might, Jesus offered a significant sigh and used a Greek formulation for open up. Another problem apparently solved. From that moment on, Jesus, by popular acclaim, had become someone who 'even makes the deaf hear and the dumb speak'.

But hearing loss, in this as in so many contexts, emerges time and again as the poor relation among the disabilities. Thus, there is no mention of the deaf among the lame, the halt and the blind. In Shakespeare's *As You Like It*, when the melancholy Jaques enumerates the characteristics of the seven ages of man, he conspicuously omits to give a name to deafness. 'Last scene of all,' he muses,

> That ends this strange, eventful history,
> Is second childishness and mere oblivion,
> Sans teeth, sans eyes, sans taste, sans everything . . .

Speech loss in early Christian times is given almost mystical status, and the origin of speech itself, as well as the seeming lack of it, are seen once again as matters for spiritual contemplation. In the New Testament Zachariah has his speechlessness directly attributed to his lack of faith. From the very first, it seems (according to the early Christians), there was a divinely decreed ascending order in a creature's communicative ability – from the cow to the parrot up to the human being. (Perhaps it was from this time that the word dumb became directly associated with deafness and took on its pejorative meaning.)

Where Justinian was trying in his own legalistic way to change these attitudes, only two centuries after his code was published it was the Christian teachers who were once again muscling in. The Venerable Bede, for example, writing in his monk's cell in the north-east of England in the eighth century, declared that being unable to speak was something of theological rather than physical concern. But then he told how in the preceding century a speechless boy had been referred to Bishop John of Hexham for help. The bishop, following the procedures attributed to Jesus, asked the boy to stick out his tongue, which he did, and then made the sign of the cross, before asking the boy to say words after him. The boy did as he was told, and – improbably or not! – he was declared cured, and another insurmountable problem had apparently been solved. On the other hand, it was subsequently disclosed that the skin problem, with which the same boy was also afflicted and which took the form of scabs on his hairless head, had to be referred to a local doctor.

And not only the Christians got in on the act. A century ahead of Bede the Prophet Muhammad, now the acknowledged spiritual leader to 800 million Muslims, claimed to have been visited by the Angel Gabriel and to have been told by him that he, Muhammad, was the messenger of God. This led Muhammad to devote his life to religious contemplation and to give close attention to the poor and the disabled, including the blind and the deaf. His teachings were taken up with zeal two hundred years after his death by thinking Muslims who spoke in terms of 'impairment', 'curtailment' and 'complete loss' when referring to defective sight and hearing – although, as it turned out, they also tended to give more attention to the blind than they did to those with hearing loss. At approximately the same time the hierarchy of the Roman Catholic Church was laying down its own parameters vis-à-vis deaf people. They were distinctly unambiguous. Deaf individuals continued to be denied rights of inheritance, were barred from participating in mass and were not allowed to marry.

It was a dispensation which could not last, but it was not until the twelfth century in Europe that the teachings of Aristotle and Plato were dusted down for serious reconsideration and, in the fullness of time, for some fundamental questioning. Teachers and thinkers – including religious thinkers – accepted the Aristotelian view that the soul expressed itself through the spoken word but also declared that if oralism was not for some reason possible then perhaps things could be said through the use of signs made with the hands. On the other hand, if sign language was not achievable, then the mute individual, deaf as well as dumb, would have to remain regarded – once again – as sub-human. One positive development did occur in the twelfth century: this was the papal decree that deaf individuals should be allowed to marry.

Some basic changes in attitude had come by the beginning of the sixteenth century. Teachers began to think in terms of educating the deaf without talking of souls or the involvement of miracles. Insight and enlightenment in people were possible, it now transpired, without reliance or intercession from God. In Germany, where the Protestantism of Martin Luther was gaining ground, so were the efforts (albeit isolated) to teach the deaf to speak. In Spain a monk called Pedro Ponce de Leon reached a new milestone when he started teaching small groups of deaf children the rudiments of reading and writing as well as speaking. He was favoured by the interest taken in his work by the King of Spain and influential members of the Court.

An influential textbook on how to teach the deaf to read, drawing extensively on some of de Leon's methods – and some say it was downright plagiarizing – was compiled by one Juan Pablo Bonet and published in Madrid in 1620. To illustrate his arguments he included a series of hand signals, or 'hand shapes' as they were called, to represent the letters of the alphabet. He also placed a special emphasis on the possibilities of lip-reading. The teacher, he pointed out, should be in good light so that the learner gets a clear view of the lip movements. But, more important, he insisted that the learner should be treated as a normal human being who was capable of being helped.

Bonet's enlightenment – or was it de Leon's? – influenced other treatments of the deaf which were being tried at the time. One involved purging the patient, shaving the crown of the head and massaging the area twice a day with a previously boiled mixture of spirits, saltpetre and oil from bitter almonds. (Echoes here of the Culpeper way of thinking.) This part of the patient's head would then be spoken to directly and the result, it was announced, was that 'the deaf-mute hears with clarity the voice that in no way could be heard through the ears'.

A sixteenth-century Flemish anatomist called Andreas Vesalius was a devoutly religious man but a trail-blazing radical in matters of the human body. He rejected the traditional thinking that was prevalent at the time and was heavily criticized, but not by a contemporary Italian physician, Geronimo Mercuriali, who argued that speechlessness could come from brain injury and that a child who could not hear could be helped through the stimulation of other parts of the body. The old proposition that thought, or even the soul itself, was unachievable or could not exist without speech was losing credibility.

Britain's turbulent seventeenth century saw a diverse and sometimes significant flurry of interest and research into hearing matters. John

Wilkins, a founder member of the Royal Society, wrote copiously on the development and use of language, including sign language, as a means of communicating knowledge. In one paper he cited a Turkish emperor who had his own group of mute advisers with whom he discussed private business when he did not want others to understand, using what Wilkins called a 'dialogue of gestures'. Wilkins argued the case for a greater use of 'postures' of the hands and fingers, and some of the signs he advocated are still in use today. John Bulwer, a contemporary of Wilkins, set out to prove that a person born deaf and dumb could be taught to hear the sound of words through his eyes. Although he is not known to have taught any deaf people himself, he claimed that what he called 'the language of the hand' was 'natural in all men'.

But it fell to a mathematician, John Wallis, who had apparently read Bonet's book, to come up with an alphabet of signs which, although devised three centuries ago, would be extraordinarily familiar to signers in Britain today. His view was that where speech was not effective then 'little actions and gestures' should be used instead. Each letter could be 'designed' by the positioning of the finger, the hand or another part of the body. By the time of his death he had been widely discredited as an academic who 'steals feathers from others to adorn his own cap', but his finger spelling was nevertheless being acclaimed as the quickest means of interaction and communication between deaf individuals. An associate of Wilkins, William Holder, who was one of Wallis's detractors, expanded horizons still further by introducing a new and greater emphasis on lip-reading.

Although these developments meant that people with impaired hearing were being used as the equivalent of laboratory guinea-pigs, it was important that they were also being seen as individuals as capable as anyone of thinking for themselves. Where previously mysticism and even total scepticism had prevailed some real humanity was creeping in, with an emphasis on what was possible and practicable. In the generations that followed, demand for education was such that special schools were established, one of the most notable being the Academy for the Deaf and Dumb in Edinburgh, founded in 1760 by Thomas Braidwood. He announced that within three years he would be able to teach 'anyone of a tolerable genius' to speak and read distinctly. Although it was known that he also

resorted to signing and finger spelling, he seems to have been pathologi-
cally secretive by nature and tended to keep other methods to himself
and his closest associates. But there were more positive developments
elsewhere.

At the same time there were crucial and apparently much more sophisticated developments in France and Germany. During the eighteenth
century Charles Michel de l'Epée, a priest as well as a lawyer, was to give
over much of his life to the education of children who were poor as well as
deaf. Unlike Braidwood he was not secretive and threw open his doors to a
curious public to demonstrate how his charges could reproduce whole sentences in more than one language in answer to signed questions. A dozen
years after his death de l'Epée was being acclaimed as 'the greatest of all
human creatures', and a play was written and performed to honour his
achievements. Although he was to have many followers and disciples – and
not a few detractors (and not only in France) – he remained reluctant
towards the end of his life to acknowledge that deaf people could be
capable of the same achievements as hearing people.

There followed a proliferation of new schools in Britain and conti-
nental Europe, and great strides were taken in assimilating the deaf into
society at large. The new establishments also excited an acquisitive
interest from visiting Americans, led most notably by the Reverend
Thomas Gallaudet and his supporters. But these Americans, it seems,
were treated with some very considerable reserve by the teachers they
tried to meet and to learn from in Britain, including Braidwood. Not
daunted, they headed for France, where they were able to meet and to
exchange fruitful and constructive ideas with followers of the irrepressible de l'Epée.

These developments did not mean, however, that God did not linger,
in the wings as it were, to play some more decisive parts in the reasoning
behind the teaching, if not in the teaching itself. Missionaries and the
new teachers began to join forces, convinced that their less than equivo-
cal theological methods were the most appropriate means by which they
could assist deaf people spiritually and morally. The result was that the
balance shifted back for a while to the medieval and that, once again, the
saving of souls became for a while as important in many centres as the
informed teaching of new and relatively scientific communication skills.

An undercurrent in what was otherwise a period of steady progress for the hearing impaired led to the controversy, already touched upon, which surfaced in the mid nineteenth century between the pro- and the anti-signers. Where teachers like Wilkins and de l'Epée had been enthusiasts for the development of sign languages, seeing them as a means to achieve a 'perfect language', there were also vociferous critics, who were complaining that while sign language might well make the user understood by 'savage tribes' it was hardly adequate for exchanges with bourgeois Europeans. This undercurrent became the mainstream at the 1880 conference in Milan, when the vote was carried to release deaf people from what one delegate called the 'slavery to silence' which the use of sign language would allegedly impose on them. The American delegation voted against the resolution, and within a few stormy decades it was American teachers who were at the forefront of sign language reasserting itself. But this reassertion was only possible after sign language had fallen so far out of favour that many of the professors who taught it and many of the schools at which they were employed had been obliged to cease working.

One redoubtable figure who had little sympathy with the predicament of such professors was Alexander Graham Bell, the inventor of the telephone and of gadgets for the deaf, who sought to end the use of sign language once and for all. He declared at one point that the deaf were effectively mentally retarded. But sign language, in its various forms, had supporters, covert and overt, in some unexpected places. Robert Louis Stevenson, whose book *Treasure Island* came out three years after Milan, is said to have given dictation using the finger alphabet. Both Queen Victoria and her sometime prime minister William Gladstone were said to have used sign language when communicating with deaf people.

A parallel social development during the nineteenth century was the trend towards the education of deaf individuals ceasing to be a matter of charity or the Church and becoming more an accepted responsibility for the State. But it was only one trend among many. Local benefactors were still called upon to give voluntary contributions to bolster such funds as were forthcoming from central and local government. It was at this time – the beginning of the twentieth century – that pressure groups, led by the British Deaf Association, emerged to lobby Whitehall to provide increased funds. The groups had an uphill task. Although it was a time when earphones and transmitters were beginning to be patented as a means of improving the teaching of hearing, it was also a time when deaf children could be, and still were, certified under the terms of the Mental Deficiency Bill of 1913.

A new sophistication of approach was starting to emerge and, with the increased production of popular newspapers and journals and the advertising spaces that they included, the scope was growing for new treatments and cures from less scrupulous individuals who were neither churchmen nor teachers. The superstition and mysticism that had been inherent in so many attitudes and in the treatment of people with hearing problems was making way, in the new technological age, for all sorts of quackery and humbuggery. The ethos behind this sort of thinking persists in the twenty-first century. 'A new hearing aid has been introduced for pensioners,' says a piece of paper, which fell out of a magazine I was reading the other day. 'The effect is immediate. No fuss, no bother.' And the smaller print? 'The sound is crisp and clear and you will be astonished just how easily conversations, television or radio can be heard with such a small device . . . If you already wear a hearing aid', it adds, 'you will be interested . . . Simply complete the form overleaf . . . The information pack is free, without any obligation.' You have to tick the little box if you are a pensioner, and, of course, no postage stamp is required.

Then there is the postcard, which may be found on empty seats on public transport, or again, falling out of respectable magazines and newspapers. It is illustrated with a photomontage of a man in the mandatory white coat climbing off the top of a step-ladder into a gigantic ear – enough to give a delicate soul scope for a nightmare. Overleaf, you are offered a free copy of what it declares (on what basis?) is 'the best-selling book' *Five Steps to Better Hearing* if you fill in the appropriate spaces with your name, address and telephone number. Once again, no postage stamp is required, and, once again, you tick the little box if you are a retired person.

Or you may be seduced by the *Readers' Digest Family Guide to Alternative Medicine*, published in 1991. The *Readers' Digest*, after all, is one of the world's most widely read publications and is readily found in any self-respecting doctor's waiting-room – perhaps even at some audiology clinics. The family guide, on the other hand, is a big coffee-table book. It is one you may perhaps consult – and on page 106, under the heading 'Deafness', you will read that 'practitioners' (unspecified) believe that diet can affect the functioning of the ears. Vitamins A (which comes in cheese, eggs, liver and carrots) and B1 (which comes in brewer's yeast – does that mean beer? – wholemeal bread, potatoes and peanuts) are said to help repair damaged cell tissue and to strengthen the auditory nerve. 'Ah, but', said a learned academic in the hearing field when I mentioned this to him, 'this is very dubious, you know.'

Advice on the true usefulness and validity of offers such as these, when you ask for it from NHS or local authority specialists, is guarded, although one lip-reading teacher I know said she wouldn't touch the offer of 'a new hearing aid for pensioners' with a barge-pole. Opinions from her and from experienced fellow lip-readers on the equipment offered inevitably come in the form of a reserved judgement. So how is the innocent but needy person able to have confidence in such offers? What, you may ask, has changed in, say, the last hundred years? Has any measurable difference been made by the Trade Descriptions Act, under the terms of which items traded must do what the packaging promises they will do?

You can, of course, go to the Hearing Aid Council, which spends much of its time dealing with complaints and which knows a lot about hearing aids and the people who deal in them. Or you can phone the RNID helpline, which is very keen on getting and providing consumer satisfaction. But there is, when you take a closer look, an awful lot on offer out there, and you can be forgiven if you feel perplexed or even overwhelmed by what you see. At the end of a wearing and unfulfilling day you may still be left wondering, as I am, that if these are the approved – or apparently approved – selling tactics aimed at the gullible in the twenty-first century, how far have we actually advanced since the first highly questionable methods were employed a century ago?

At that time there were, in fact, a dedicated handful of shrewd individuals on the job, determined to root out what smelled like malpractice and undeterred by whatever rules of slander or libel may have been in operation at the time. The little books they published following their investigations are difficult to track down nowadays, but when you do find them they are full of information, which remains to this day as depressing as it is revealing. Some examples of their findings follow.

Primus inter pares of the ferrets who were determined to nail these malpractitioners and fraudsters was a man called Evan Yellon, who seems to have lived in Hertfordshire and who, at the beginning of the twentieth century, was honorary director of the British and Foreign Deaf Association (which no longer exists) and also the editor of *The Albion*, a journal aimed at deaf readers. In the USA, where at this time there was a great deal of public activity – serious as well as fraudulent – to help people with hearing loss, he was accorded noteworthy status by the American Medical Association (AMA) among others.

In a little book called *Deafness Cure Fakes*, published in Chicago in 1914, the AMA described Mr Yellon as a journalist of the militant type. 'Himself a sufferer from deafness, he appreciates the viciousness of the victimization carried on by the deafness-cure quacks. While a layman, Mr Yellon expresses himself with no uncertainty regarding the dangers of what he (slightly inaccurately) sees as quackery.' And then the AMA quotes from Yellon's own book, *Surdus in Search of His Hearing* (1906), on what Yellon calls 'the very world of distinction' between the qualified specialist and the quack. (*Surdus* is the latin for deaf.)

'In the quack', Yellon wrote, 'we have in the majority of cases a man who does not possess even a sound general education, and very often who does not understand the elements of ordinary personal cleanliness ... He is a man moving in the dark, and thus making only blind shots ... A man of mysterious methods and secret remedies, and his vogue today is at once a significant token and, as I have said, a menace to the community.'

The AMA, in its enthusiasm, described the British Isles as 'that verdant field for medical fakers' (among whom it unhesitatingly included quacks known to be of American origin). But it also warily pointed out that while Yellon's words had been directed against those who operated in the British Isles, they could be applied 'with equal truth and equal force' to those American fakers who claimed to be selling deafness cures.

Yellon himself, in his original Surdus book, said he was offering 'a guide for that section of the public so long victimized by fakes and humbugs, the deaf'. Anyone knowing anything about the ear, he said, would understand 'the downright mad folly' involved in any attempt by the unqualified and unskilled to treat an ear ailment. Even to fill in and submit a diagnosis form for treatment from a man probably not possessing an atom of knowledge about the ear was insane.

Surdus, in his exploratory search for better hearing, makes a series of pilgrimages to a handful of consulting-rooms at what seem to be quality addresses in central London. The addresses are not always what they seem. The reception areas are single rooms, sometimes 'smart sitting-rooms' but sometimes barely furnished spaces above a shop or above a railway ticket office. At Marble Arch he found the consulting physician was himself 'away, ill'; at Amberley House in the Strand the director was also 'away' but had left instructions to would-be patients to fill in the form and leave their money; at a Bloomsbury address the doctor was absent 'in America'; at Holborn, after hammering on a locked door, he learned that the 'professor' was momentarily 'out' and 'could not be found'; and so on.

When he could not get a one-to-one consultation Yellon wrote to one of the more promising providers, sending in the mandatory form from several different addresses, listing in each case widely differing symptoms. In each case his reply contained the same diagnosis and the same prescription to take the same lotion and wear the same ear-pads, wetted with another prescribed solution, for half an hour each night before going to bed. Another provider offered what he called 'disguised' aids, in the form of acoustic fans, acoustic walking sticks, acoustic books and even acoustic easy chairs, 'elegantly gilded and nicely upholstered'.

At the Light Cure Institute, with consulting-rooms just off Eaton Square, the clientele was probably better off than those going to Holborn or Oxford Street. Here the basis of the treatment was electricity in various forms: there was the light of ultra-violet rays to stimulate and improve the quality of the blood around the ears; vibration to loosen bones in the same area; currents to pass through the body and strengthen the auditory nerve; and there was an 'electro-chemical ear bath' to wash away unwanted sediments and deposits from the ears. Would-be clients were advised that when there was no reply from the Eaton Square address they should write to the director at his country residence in Buckinghamshire.

One or two of the providers seem to have had an inkling of likely trends in the real world. While offering trumpets for five guineas (£5.25, or several hundred pounds at today's prices) and 'very elaborate' moulded ear pieces for ten times as much, they did acknowledge that trends might be in a different direction. An invisible aid, it was agreed, would probably come one day, but, as Yellon himself pointed out, 'it is a dream of the remote future', adding that 'a fair fortune awaits its lucky inventor'.

But how ingenious and how successful in the great American market place were those manufacturers and others whom the AMA unhesitatingly described as the American fakers? Their tones as they relayed these descriptions were much more damning than those proffered by the comparatively gentleman-like Evan Yellon. The reason, one suspects, is that Yellon was circumscribed to some extent by the much more stringent prevailing British libel laws. The laws in this area were different in the USA, and the possibility of suing in the courts was that much less.

The devices described indicated a different sort of lateral thinking when it came to hearing loss. In discussing products of the so-called Actina Appliance Company, Kansas, the author noted that 'magnetic' and 'electric' developments in Britain were dismissed by the company as 'nonsense'. In most cases of deafness what was needed was clearances of the 'blockages', which could be achieved by inhaling a mixture of oil of mustard and oil of sassafras held in a small steel vial with screw caps at each end. The cost (in the 1890s) was $10; the smell on unpacking the device was, according to the AMA, worth $10 to get away from.

The AMA also looked at the claims of one 'Dr' George Coutant, who, without any real qualifications, after a period operating from premises also used by companies offering cures for drunkenness and for baldness, set up shop on New York's Broadway. 'It is far from my nature and disposition to boast,' Coutant told inquirers, 'and if I had not been a physician [sic] I would have been a clergyman. I am inherently conscientious . . . I know the only satisfactory method of treating deafness.' His method was to sell, for up to $10 a package, five small boxes of pills, a small tin of salve, a nasal douche and some nickel-plated tubing that, said the AMA, smelled like decayed onion. Two weeks after delivery of this package a further letter from Coutant urges the customer not to look for 'miracles' and to maintain 'calm perseverance' and informing him, in the sweetest, most duplicitous way possible, that more money was required for further treatment. Coutant, the AMA concluded, had no professional standing and was a 'swindler'.

A third concern examined by the AMA was the Morley Company of Philadelphia. This company produced something called the Morley Ear Phone, which consisted of a circular piece of oiled silk about quarter of an inch in diameter – an artificial eardrum – through the centre of which an anchored piece of waxed silk thread was passed to hold the silk piece in position. A small piece of flexible tubing was used to help insert the device into the ear. Once in place, the company said, it was 'more sensitive to vibration and more powerful as a sound transmitter than any other known device'. In short, it was claimed, it restored hearing 'like magic'. For the AMA the exorbitant prices and fraudulent claims were 'not merely an injury to the purse, but a distinct menace to the health of the deaf'.

And so on. Such a list could, with diligence and assiduous searching, be brought up to date. The twenty-first century has its own share of fraudsters and claimants, as well as those who may be thought to edge close to a rather grey area with boasts that they sell, for instance, 'the world's finest hearing aids'. In a letter received in early 2003 from a company with more than fifty branches nationwide I was told that 'a while ago' I had inquired about the 'fantastic' range of hearing aids available. As a consequence I had an appointment for 2 p.m. for the following 23 June, which I could confirm either in writing or by free phone call on the company's 'priority appointment' line. I am still thinking about it . . .

Another offer, this time of cash, is one to which I have devoted rather less thought. One Monday in August 2003 I received a personal letter (Dear Mr Simmons, etc.) from a smart address in central London which opened with: 'As promised, we hereby officially confirm your definite entitlement to tax-free cash in our new, free £250,000 cash-match draw with your lucky number . . . You will definitely receive a cash award or may even be a major cash prize winner, Mr Simmons . . . No purchase is needed . . . We are bound to stick to our word!' On reading these lines I felt like invoking the spirit of Mr Yellon, wherever he was, or the AMA to investigate. The tone, after all, was very familiar.

But that was not all. At the end of the same week I received another letter from the same smart address which was much more exhortatory in tone. 'Dear Mr Simmons,' it started, 'Have you claimed your tax-free cash? I sincerely hope you have, but if you have not there is still time!' And it ended: 'Claim the money you are *definitely* entitled to!' And what, you may ask, was it all about? Answer: Health insurance, protecting me, said the small print, against 'the real risks' in life, such as – wait for it – injury resulting in 'total loss of eyesight, hearing, speech, paralysis'. Nothing about hearing impairment as such, only more cajoling. 'What might your lucky number have won ... ?'

I will, alas, never know.

SIX

The company you keep

THERE CAN BE a strange eloquence about people who have hearing loss, in which, ironically, their ability to hear or speak plays no part. You seem to recognize them when you see them. Try, for example, when, as a hearing person, you meet someone whom you know has hearing problems to pause for a less than courteous moment to look at their eyes. Or if you have access to illustrated books about deaf people study the photographs of them and look, once again, at the eyes: that is where the eloquence comes in. There is a piercing, searching look of concentration about them, a look that tells you they are constantly in need of a focus through which to understand more clearly what is going on around them.

This exercise applies most particularly to those individuals who have acknowledged there is a hearing problem. Not acknowledging means there may well be an evasiveness about the eyes! But then not everyone is able to own up, and one of the surprising things about losing your hearing in later life is the change you detect in long-standing friends and acquaintances when you tell them you cannot hear as well as once you did. It quickly becomes clear – in a covert sort of way, for it is not something to be shouted from the rooftops – that you may have more in common than either of you has previously been willing to admit. 'Oh,' said one friend, quite spontaneously, 'I think I must have been deaf for years . . . But I simply couldn't wear a hearing aid. On the other hand, I do keep one in my pocket just in case . . .' And, so saying, he fished into his jacket pocket and held the thing up with a faintly embarrassed and rather bent-pin smile at the distasteful procedure he was going through.

Another friend, hitherto regarded by me as a rather proud and dignified person, confided to me once she saw me wearing my hearing aid that, despite her own problem, she always made the effort to give the appearance of hearing, even in a group. However, this meant that she was also constantly saddled, she said, with the worrying concern that her mask might unexpectedly slip should someone in the group suddenly turn on her and ask her views on what had just been said, even though she hadn't heard. This person had to be commended, at the very least, for her new-found willingness to share her secret and to be honest. The more usual reaction, but one of more questionable honesty, is to resort to a sort of defence mechanism, to admit that hearing loss may have occurred, or that it may be coming, and then to add, with a nervous semi-nudge, 'But, of course, I manage.'

Statistical facts offer their own perverse comfort. Hearing loss, say the specialists, is the most common sensory disability in the developed world. Whatever their feelings, the fact is that the deaf and the hearing impaired, taken all together, are not alone. Far from it. In Britain, at the beginning of the twenty-first century it was estimated that at least 14 per cent of the population have significant hearing difficulties. The odds of becoming one of this huge number increases markedly after the age of fifty. As many as three out of every four people with hearing problems are over sixty. And the corollary to this is that the percentage of the population over sixty is increasing dramatically.

The guilty party in an unknown number of cases seems to be a gene called BRN-3C, something which has been preoccupying Dr Sally Dawson, a researcher at University College London. With supporting funds from Help the Aged she has been exploring whether there is a genetic link involved in hearing loss. The gene under scrutiny is supposed to protect and repair the relevant cells in the inner ear, but if it ceases to function it could be because the cells have been overwhelmed by the damage they have suffered as a result of too much noise.

Consolation for those who have hearing loss – if consolation is the right word – has to be sought where it can be found. But the world which they inhabit is tough. It is tough to learn that, in most cases, hearing that is lost in later years cannot, on present knowledge, be restored through any natural process; more often than not, it cannot be cured. The possibility that the genes may be involved and the extent to which heredity may have a part to play is not something that currently appeals, as an avenue of research, to the big pharmaceutical companies. In some academic centres, there are developments in this very area, but they are probably some years away from being of benefit to the consumer.

At present, defective hearing can only be eased through the use of decidedly unnatural and electronic or electrical devices. There are the rituals and the procedures that one has to go through to get one of these devices, routines which in themselves may be seen as constituting a final push from apparent normality to abnormality. The culminating moment of these routines is being presented with a very rare item that, if it is not to be surgically screwed into your scalp or hung around your neck, has to be unceremoniously squeezed into your ear. Then, of course, if you don't want the NHS involved, there is the matter of expense.

The important consolation, however, is that some comparably ugly rituals have also been happening to other people. You can give half a cheer to the fact that hearing loss knows no boundaries of race, colour or creed and that the great and the good, as well as the recalcitrant and congenitally grumpy, are all susceptible. 'We know the words,' wrote one sufferer I read about. 'We have had a career, we have had money, family and responsibilities, and IQ tests are not necessary; we may need care and attention – sometimes – but we don't need a special education.' Even though, for centuries and until relatively recently, deafness, and especially congenital deafness, has been linked to dumbness and dumbness has frequently been linked to stupidity, it is now evident that, when hearing loss is imminent, one's level of intelligence and sensitivity generally remain intact and can do nothing to keep hearing loss at bay. Perhaps it is a blessing of sorts to know that other people have been similarly afflicted, even though very few of them have wanted to make a song or dance about it.

A number of those who have been through hearing loss have written down their experiences – more a lament than a song, and an account, often, of the shock, desperation and despair they have gone through. These individuals have described, sometimes with extraordinary eloquence, how they have sought to make the best of a bad job, reconciled to the fact in many cases that, since their condition was essentially incurable, not a lot of people have really cared. The very act of writing it all down, as these pages may be seen to testify, has been therapeutic. Almost none of the writings has expressed significant happiness about the condition being described, although, as I have mentioned earlier, I did come across that peculiar American book called *Deafness and Cheerfulness*. I did not find it very helpful.

The RNID library has drawn up its own very neat list of those it calls 'famous deaf people'. It was typed out when I last saw it and filled half a dozen sheets of A4 paper. It is international in character, drawing mainly on the developed world, and contained more than 250 names from the sixteenth-century French poet Pierre Ronsard onwards to Kate Adie, the BBC's very twenty-first century broadcaster. It did not differentiate between the degree of deafness affecting the individuals, which meant that without laborious research it was not always possible to know which of them had the age-related condition that is my main concern. All manner of individuals were included, but it did not take much searching to find names that were conspicuously missing. Jack Straw, for example, who was foreign secretary when the Tony Blair government became deeply embroiled in Iraq, was not there; nor was Nelson Mandela, the charismatic former president and political prisoner of South Africa, who is well into his eighties and has hearing loss; nor, for that matter, was Deng Xiaoping, the one-time post-Mao reformist leader of the People's Republic of China. The list is long.

But the list repays study, and some interesting facts immediately become apparent. The first striking point is that a high proportion of those listed distinguished themselves as artists or architects. Their profile is high alongside that of the politicians, sportsmen, inventors, missionaries, composers, university lecturers and business people who are also there in abundance. Nor is this the only such list. Other organizations and people have drawn up lists of their own, sometimes coming up with rather different results. One, originating in the USA, chooses to underline the presence of a surprisingly high number of engineers and mathematicians as well as architects. Professionals acknowledge that deaf children tend to shine at mathematics, and one reason for this, according to the neurologist Oliver Sacks, is that these are people who have a great facility in picturing and thinking in what he calls 'three-dimensional space'. Their hearing capability is not their most important equipment.

It would be easy to fill a separate book with the names and the corroborative details of eminent deaf and hard-of-hearing people. What follows is necessarily very selective and very subjective. Those names that I have chosen are here mainly because they show the unexpected variety of contexts in which deafness or hearing loss has been encountered, grappled with and, in some circumstances, actually overcome.

TOP PEOPLE

Royal family members (including some in the present British royal family) have suffered from hearing impairment, sometimes through heredity, although they and statesmen and leading politicians have developed their own distinctive ways of coping. The majority choose or have chosen, for obvious reasons, not to dwell on the matter. You could say that Nelson Mandela belongs to this category; he has barely acknowledged, even to his authorized biographer, the fact of hearing loss, although he has conceded that the use of a hearing aid brings its own disciplines. And he has publicly declared that for effective communication, which he should know all about, when you have such a disability you need 'the understanding, expertise, love and dedication' of many people. His poor hearing has been with him at least since the mid-1990s.

At the other extreme Adolf Hitler, at the height of his powers as leader of the Third Reich, was a sufferer. Tinnitus is believed to have affected him in his early forties and was probably brought on by his own stressful decisions – such as, according to some theories, the so-called Night of the Long Knives (29–30 June 1934), when he authorized the liquidation of several hundred military and political rivals. Ten years later came the bomb attempt on his own life, led by Count von Stauffenberg when the Second World War was at its most intense. This resulted in a perforated ear drum.

Winston Churchill, between fulminating against Hitler, incurred hearing loss while he was still on the front bench, as Leader of the Opposition in the House of Commons. Socially, he would employ numerous tactics to disguise his disability, one of which was to talk endlessly across those people – such as dinner guests and diplomats, as well as troublesome politicians! – in whose company he found himself. In the Commons, this was not a tactic he could easily employ, so – using the tactic we've seen employed by the novelist Evelyn Waugh – he would resort, much to the consternation of some and the amusement of others, to removing ostentatiously his hearing aid during speeches he did not want to hear and conspicuously placing it on the Dispatch Box in front of him.

Defeat in the General Election of 1945, after a successful leadership during the war, hit Churchill hard, and defeat in the election that followed in 1950, in his seventy-sixth year, hit him even harder. Although he gave all he could as the Opposition leader, his inner circle was well aware that hearing loss troubled him increasingly. His family knew well that he resented having to use his hearing aid and, to the exasperation of everyone around him, he would frequently refuse to use one at all. Towards the end of his life he became withdrawn and would go for hours on end not speaking to anyone and apparently not hearing others when they were speaking to him. His daughter, Mary Soames, was to record later that he increasingly grew to hate being alone, even though in fact he rarely was. His widow Clementine, ennobled to the House of Lords after his death, was an avid attender at debates until she, too, was to lose her hearing two years after her husband's death. By the end of her life, in echoes of what had gone before, she, too, was withdrawing, as her late husband had done, into what her daughter Mary called 'great and distant silences'.

Nor have American presidents been immune. Bill Clinton, like the late Ronald Reagan before him, both apparently did wonders to promote the cause of hearing-loss sufferers when they publicly acknowledged their own hearing problems. The cause in Clinton's case is commonly thought to have been his excessive zeal in playing the saxophone in a band during his teens. According to a *New York Times* report (3 October 1997), hearing had presented him with significant problems even since the early 1980s when he was Governor of the State of Arkansas. By 1997 he was having difficulty hearing people in crowded rooms and even, when he was speech-making, in hearing hecklers. The loss had nothing to do with short-term political opportunism. The diagnosis was high-frequency hearing loss in both ears, typical of the sort of loss that comes with ageing and with a previous exposure to loud noise. I wrote to Clinton for first-hand details; his office wrote back saying that his memoirs had precedence but that he appreciated my interest and sent his best wishes! 'We are probably the world's greatest power – in hearing aids,' a tongue-in-cheek American friend wrote to me in June 2004.

One of the most revealing accounts of suddenly becoming deaf – as opposed to acquiring hearing loss – is that written by Jack Ashley. He was an MP thought to have a promising ministerial career in front of him but who became deaf in the winter of 1967. 'I thought I had known despair,' he wrote, 'but now I felt a chill and a deeper sadness, as if part of me was dead . . . I felt in my heart that I had begun a life of tomb-like silence.' Within a few days of this new dismal beginning he took his first walk, with his wife Pauline, through his Lancashire constituency. 'It was', he said, 'the bleakest stroll of my life.' His first deaf experience of the perpetually noisy Commons division lobby was that the place, which was normally one of intrigue and whispered confidences among MPs, had become one of the world's loneliest places. One of his first reactions was that the confident, easy-going relationships with people, which he had always taken for granted, were gone for ever. He could also say goodbye to a glittering career.

Ashley found that the intense loneliness that comes, however briefly, to almost everyone who experiences sudden hearing loss was deeply traumatic. 'I was cut off from mankind,' he wrote, 'surrounded by an invisible, impenetrable barrier. I could see people clearly, but they belonged to a different world – a world of talk, of music and laughter.' But Jack Ashley was a person of amazing resilience. Once he had tasted the isolation he acquired a new strength in his determination to end it by throwing himself into campaigning on behalf of others. Deaf people, he announced, were commonly regarded as second-class citizens, and he quickly decided it was not right that blind people, for example, were getting twenty times more charitable donations than those who were deaf. In 1986 he and his wife founded the Hearing Research Trust, a body now better known as Defeating Deafness, which supports academic research into all sorts of esoteric areas. A spokesperson of stature had arrived.

But campaigning has been no walkover. 'Helping deaf people,' Ashley noted nearly twenty years after going deaf, 'and attempting to communicate with them, is a laudable endeavour. It must, nevertheless, be carefully watched because it can so easily become patronizing. It is not easy to accept the fact that some people look down on the deaf, but it is so. They tend to equate loss of hearing with loss of reason, perhaps because of the invisibility of the handicap or a result of difficulty in communicating.

It is one of the heaviest burdens that deaf people have to bear.' In addition to playing a leading role in the advancement of hearing research, Ashley was to become patron or president or non-executive chairman of a number of organizations associated with deafness or hearing loss.

Another hearing-impaired former MP, who was a contemporary of Jack Ashley, is the Rt Hon. Tony Benn. He was born with a hereditary right to a seat in the House of Lords but fought to have the law changed so that he could become a member of the House of Commons. In the three-year spell which I enjoyed in the mid-1960s as a parliamentary journalist sitting in the Commons Press Gallery I was able to watch his usually impeccable and often witty performances as Minister for Aviation and, later, for Minister for Technology. One of the great achievements during his tenure was the launch of Concorde, the noisiest (!) and the most elegant aircraft to grace the skies. On his retirement from the Commons in 2001 he publicly and characteristically announced his determination to become an even more explicitly political animal on platforms up and down the country. At about the same time he chose to launch himself as a *de facto* campaigner for people with hearing loss. When I wrote asking him for some thoughts on his experience that he might share with me for the purposes of this book, he wrote back by return of post.

'I'm not really deaf in a serious way,' he said, 'but my hearing is bad enough to miss out a lot of what I hear in conversation and also I can't enjoy the movies or the theatre because I just don't pick up the dialogue as well as I should.' He had discovered he was deaf at a crowded meeting in a schoolroom in his Bristol constituency – after a ten-minute interchange with a man he assumed was a heckler but who was in fact justdesperately pleading for a window to be opened to get some fresh air. 'That is how I got my NHS hearing aids,' he went on, 'but they whistle and buzz or go dead and are not as effective as they could be.' He told me that he hadn't, as a matter of principle, paid for a private digital aid, 'but it would be lovely if they were available on the NHS.' (Within weeks of this letter the government indicated that something approximating to this loveliness was on its way, and such aids would be universally available within a few years.)

Tony Benn's rather quirky methods of caring for his hearing aids are not recommended. 'On one occasion', he wrote, 'I took them out of my ears just as I dropped off to sleep and accidentally put them in a cup of cold tea – which seemed to improve them slightly. On other occasions I have left them in my shirt pocket and they have been through the washing machine, which also seems to help!' On a more serious note, he suggested that the important thing was not to be shy about deafness: 'If I see someone with hearing aids, I always ask about them, inquire whether they work properly, and I find it gives deaf people a boost to know that you understand.'

Michael Foot, a veteran parliamentarian and polemicist, announced in 2004, in his ninety-first year, that he had never worried much about his health, even though he knew he wouldn't still be alive if it weren't for the NHS. But he did acknowledge, although not quite explicitly, that he had hearing problems, saying that he had had a hearing aid fitted three or four years previously. He noted with some glee that he could still talk on the telephone without the aid, but added, 'Not being able to do my hearing aids properly is my only imbecility.'

At the end of 2002 the Foreign Office organized an event of its own dedicated to the discussion and promotion of deaf issues. Public acknowledgement was given to the contributions to foreign policy made by deaf and hard-of-hearing Foreign Office staff. Jack Straw, foreign secretary, who lost his hearing in one ear some years ago and is also known to suffer from tinnitus, said pointedly that he was well aware of the difficulties that come with hearing loss. 'But', he said, 'this is hardly an insurmountable barrier, and with the right investment in training, deaf and hard-of-hearing staff can integrate seamlessly into any team.' The Foreign Office, he announced with some paternal pride, was setting standards for 'the rest of Whitehall' to follow.

The upper classes, clinging, perhaps, to stiff-upper-lip syndrome, tend to keep their hearing problems to themselves. One nineteenth-century aristocrat who didn't was Lord Lytton, novelist and sometime minister in Disraeli's government. He was a prolific and successful writer – completing *The Last Days of Pompeii* when he was thirty – but such a bad speaker that his fellow Parliamentarians and others could barely understand him. Questioners addressing him as a minister would frequently have to wait a day or more for their answers because he had to read their words first in Hansard before he could formulate a coherent reply.

MUSICIANS

There is something especially haunting about the fact that musicians – men and women who derive satisfaction and who may earn a living from creating beautiful sounds – should be subjected to hearing loss or deafness. Beethoven, for example, clearly felt himself very much alone and was deeply depressed when he was hit in this way in his early thirties. He tried occasionally to make the most of it – 'Let your deafness be no longer a secret, even in art,' he said – but he spent a great deal of time torturing himself, thinking himself alone in his affliction, although he obviously was not. Perhaps he was of his time. Evelyn Glennie – whom I have already mentioned and will discuss shortly – the Scottish-born percussionist who currently enjoys world-wide acclaim despite being deaf. She has described her ability 'to talk to people through music' as a source of great happiness. But the piquancy of the predicament of a musician who is deaf cannot be overstated.

Beethoven was a familiar figure in the early nineteenth century in Heiligenstadt, which was then a pleasant village on the outskirts of Vienna. It offered him a series of bolt-holes when he came to the village, as he often did, to escape the rigours and the demands of the city – many of them self-imposed – and in order to give himself sufficient space to devote time to contemplation and yet more composition. But, however idyllic his surroundings, his deteriorating hearing made him suspicious, even paranoid, and if he thought someone was prying on him or his music-making he would immediately take steps to move on to another bolt-hole in the neighbourhood.

His frequent visits to the village in his mid-twenties must have included therapeutic moments. Heiligenstadt was then surrounded by vineyards and was distinctly rural in character – although later, as it became urbanized, it became a hotbed of political revolution. For Beethoven ears were not the only problem. The need for him to beat a retreat there came at a pivotal time. There had been a number of tempestuous episodes in his love life, and Vienna's concert-goers, both those who were enthusiastic for his less-than-orthodox ways of music-making as well as those who were more critical, were beginning to encroach on his space.

Towards the end of the eighteenth century, when he was still not halfway through his life, he first noticed that he could not clearly hear high-pitched ounds and was unable to make sense of what he, in his increasing irascibility, decided – as many others do – was the extraordinary mumbling of the person with whom he was talking. He himself attributed his loss to a bout of typhus or perhaps to some undefined stomach troubles. Others, less charitable, suggested dysentery or tuberculosis (to which the family was susceptible) or even some form of venereal disease. Twentieth-century researchers have suggested otosclerosis or Paget's disease. But, whatever the cause, it was unavoidable and irreversible. Furthermore, he still had a mountain to climb in terms of musical output. At this point he had composed only two of his nine symphonies and only two of his five piano concertos. His greatest works were yet to come.

Sitting alone in one of his village hideaways he wrote his famous 'Heiligenstadt Testament', articulating what his deafness meant to him, a creative artist in the business, through his music, of communicating. It makes heart-rending reading. 'Oh, my fellow men who consider me or describe me as unfriendly, peevish or misanthropic,' he writes, 'how greatly do you wrong me. How humiliated I have felt to have someone standing at my side who can hear the distant sound of the flute, and I have heard nothing . . .' It is small wonder, he admits, that he has been driven to despair, even to the point of contemplating suicide, and 'the only thing that held me back was my art'.

He had dragged on 'this miserable existence', he said, because he had to, and he pleaded with those who were closest to him not to give away his secret and to tell anyone who was over-curious that he was merely getting absent-minded. In desperation he tried several pointless remedies, and the exasperation he went through can only be imagined. And the thought of trying some of the treatments, so called, which were available at this time must have depressed him no end. There were water shocks and other shocks mechanically induced, and there was the revolving chair, which could turn the patient a hundred times a minute, leading to blood pouring from the nose and the ears and a loss of consciousness. Those he did try included a supervised submersion in the River Danube, a cold bath and the application of ointment to different parts of his body, as well as a range of different ear trumpets, all to no avail. His own solution was to place one end of a piece of wood on the vibrating surface of a piano and to hold the other end between his teeth. In this way, he declared, he could 'hear' sounds as they were being made.

The composer wrote that he was accompanied now everywhere he went by the 'ghost' or the 'demon' of his inadequate hearing. One of his remedies – which will be familiar to millions with hearing loss – was to avoid unnecessary contact with people. Tragically, he more or less stopped performing in public, although when he did perform it was with even more boldness than usual. His output as a composer became more and more idiosyncratic as he began to express emotions in his music in a way they had not been expressed before. Now there was pain as well as triumph, sorrow as well as joy, all coming out in what musicologists describe as mysterious harmonies.

When his music was performed he continued to have experiences of almost unbearable poignancy. On one occasion, conducting a rehearsal for his only opera, *Fidelio*, he kept losing track of what the (inaudible) orchestra was actually playing and which words were being sung. When the discrepancies were pointed out to him, his humiliating confusion was such that he had to abandon the session and leave the building immediately. At the end of one of the first performances of his amazing *Ninth Symphony* he was able to see, although he could not hear, the audience's wild enthusiasm for his work. He was only fifty-three at the time, and less than four years later he was dead. Shortly before he died – three days after completing his last quartet – there was a chink of daylight in his benighted world. A noisy thunderstorm awoke him from his coma. 'I shall hear in heaven,' he said, and died.

The nineteenth-century Czech composer Bedrich Smetana was three years old when Beethoven died. In 1866, when Smetana was forty-two, he had just completed one of his most popular works, the opera *The Bartered Bride*, an idyllic and uncomplicated tale of the countryside, when he complained of whistling noises and other strange sounds in his ears. Within a matter of months his condition had deteriorated to such an extent that he was adjudged completely deaf. His, too, was an affliction that, some said, had been brought on by syphilis. He was about fifty years old at the time and decided to give up all musical work – mainly conducting – other than composing.

Despite his hearing loss, and despite the poverty of his later years,

Smetana went on to produce some of his best work. Two more operas came from him, *The Kiss* and *The Secret*, within a very few years and then the patriotic cycle for which he remains extraordinarily popular even today, *My Country*. The esteem and acclamation of his admirers did not stop him from succumbing to hallucinations, fits of violence and – like Beethoven – talking occasionally of suicide. But, doggedly, he continued composing and, remarkably, was able to incorporate some of his sufferings in his work. He claimed that his first string quartet, for instance, was about 'things that tortured me' and included a passage where he sought to reproduce the sounds of the tinnitus that constantly bothered him. He died, aged sixty, in a mental hospital.

The German composer Robert Schumann, who was an early contemporary of Smetana, lived a life at least as tempestuous as Beethoven's. He survived at least two complicated love affairs and an attempted suicide before dying after two years in a private asylum to which he had been admitted at his own request. He had first reported hearing problems in his early thirties and had tinnitus for much of his adult life. By 1846, two years after reporting the first symptoms, he was assailed by what he called a constant 'roaring' in his ears.

There are a number of other prominent musicians afflicted in this way. One was the French composer Gabriel Fauré, who began to lose his hearing at about the age of sixty, at a critical juncture in his career and just when his music was increasingly being acclaimed. He said that the sounds he began to hear were so distorted that they seemed to him to be 'a veritable cacophony', and although by common consent he continued to produce what many considered master-works, he would choose to remain closeted in his own room when the applause in the concert hall was at its most intense.

The avant-garde English-born composer (of Australian parentage), Constant Lambert, was deaf in one ear for much of his life. Hearing loss became a serious matter for Ralph Vaughan Williams after what has been described as 'the bitterest disappointment of his musical life'. This was a totally unsatisfying (to him) Covent Garden production of *The Pilgrim's Progress*, a work which had taken him forty years to complete. Five years before his death, however, he was heartened enough to marry for a second time and also, in a gesture of bold eccentricity, to have his portrait painted, complete with hearing aid. Apart from deafness, said his biographer, he was in good health.

Evelyn Glennie was born in 1965 and has given – and derived – much pleasure from music-making. She argues passionately that deaf children should be introduced to music as early as possible. She learned to assert herself – through her music – by holding the loudspeakers of the stereo system she was listening to in her hands or between her knees in order to catch the beat and the vibrations of what was being played. 'Music', she says, 'comes as much from the heart as through the ears.' Playing in all parts of the world has kept her busy and preoccupied, but, as she admits in her autobiography, the reality of her disability has still occasionally caught up with her: 'I sometimes felt I was fighting a lonely and rather dispiriting battle.'

It was at the age of eight that she noticed she was having difficulty hearing – even though by then she was beginning to play the piano, the guitar, the mouth organ and the clarinet. Within a year she was also gaining distinction as an accomplished musical performer. Then, at the age of twelve, her family was advised that she attend the local school for deaf children – something she staunchly resisted in favour of the nearest academy for music, going on to the Royal Academy of Music in London at the age of seventeen. By this time she had decided that wearing hearing aids was a waste of time and concentrated on lip-reading. By 1994 she was able to tell the world, in a *Time* magazine interview, that she did not think in terms of loud or soft but in terms of the colours and emotions that come to mind as she watches the conductor and the rest of the orchestra around her.

In such a context, it is an uncomfortable fact that any loud music can cause momentary, or longer-term, hearing loss and that the most serious damage comes from prolonged or repeated exposure to what might be called the louder-the-better type of music. It is now well established that the short-term hearing loss commonly experienced after being exposed to abnormally loud music termed temporary threshold shift can ultimately develop into permanent ear damage. Amplified rock music, it is now agreed, is louder – and therefore more damaging – than a nearby helicopter in flight, than a jet aircraft taking off 500 metres away, than a pneumatic drill or a passing motor-cycle. The roll call of well-known contemporary musicians experiencing a degree of hearing loss or tinnitus is long and includes Lars Ulrich of Metallica (all members of which now wear earplugs during performance), Eric Clapton, Neil Young, Phil Collins, Sting, Bono, Huey Lewis, Ozzy Osbourne, Barbra Streisand, Ted Nugent, Todd Rungren, Jeff Beck, Dave Swarbrick, Bob Mould and Lemmy from Motörhead, to name just a few. Norm Rogers, a drummer with a group called the Cows, has told how the group's van, at the end of a gruelling European tour, was more like 'a geriatric home . . . with members of the group screaming at each other because we just couldn't hear a thing'. Pete Townsend, guitarist with the Who, was one of the first popular musicians to confirm the occupational hazard of hearing loss. By the end of 2002 he announced that his hearing had gone 'almost completely'. Beethoven would have understood.

ARTISTS AND WRITERS

Well over a quarter of the names in the RNID library list are artists, architects or sculptors. More than once it has been suggested that a deficit in one of the senses – in this case hearing – is more than compensated for by the condition of what is missed, or lacking, to other senses. The nineteenth-century French painter Frederic Peyson, who went deaf during a bout of fever when he was a small child, became celebrated for his picture *St Margaret Bringing Down the Dragon*. One critic announced that 'being himself a martyr to the rigours of fate' it had not been difficult for him [Peyson] to portray a martyr. He also added that the painter, being deprived of speech, knew only too well how to endow the saint with her own eloquent articulacy.

The Victoria and Albert Museum in London paid its own very small tribute to artists with hearing loss in the autumn of 2000, when it mounted an exhibition called 'Visual Journeys, Silent Conversations' to coincide with Deaf Awareness Week. Artefacts and paintings were selected as visual representations of conversations with the spectator – from an eighteenth-century copy of a work by Raphael to a Meissen coffee set.

The Renaissance artist Raphael was not without an interest in hearing loss. In 1507 he completed a painting which he called simply *La Murta (The Deaf Woman)* which conveys through the fixed look about the subject's eyes the distinct probability of her disability. He also employed at least one non-hearing artist, called Pinturrichio, in the team of painters engaged in the completion of important works for the Vatican. Raphael's equally distinguished contemporary Leonardo da Vinci engaged with deafness in a different way, urging his fellow artists, in their studies of hands, to pay special attention to what they actually saw when deaf people were using the manual sign language to communicate with one another.

The Spanish artist Francisco de Goya, remembered now simply as Goya, lived life to the full, took special pride in his work and would not suffer fools. The precise cause of his hearing loss, which came in the winter of 1792–3, has never been clear, although it is widely believed to have started when the carriage in which he was travelling with a lady friend, the Duchess of Alba, broke down and he insisted, despite the bitter cold, in carrying out repairs without help. This incident apart, the parallels of Goya's experience with that of Beethoven are many, including the very years in which the affliction happened as well as the very marked impact on subsequent creative activity. His hearing, his moods – already dark in character – and the very nature of his painting were never the same again.

Where previously his work had been realistic, religious in tone and occasionally satirical – but, according to some critics, 'not particularly outstanding' – it now became disturbingly infused with grotesqueness and mystical and allegorical messages. He gave more time to depicting devils, torturers and monsters, and he also became intolerant, foul-tempered and prone to fits of violence (on one occasion attacking the Duke of Wellington, who was sitting for him, with a sword). His last pictures show people apparently alienated from one another, even isolated and depressed as he was. Sometimes, he acknowledged, he would be seized by fits of rage that he did not understand himself.

Sir Joshua Reynolds, painter and first president of the Royal Academy of Art, is generally thought to have lost his hearing after falling off a horse while on holiday with friends on the Mediterranean island of Minorca. He himself suggested, in a more impressive and possibly romanticized version, that it had been brought on by a severe cold he caught in Rome when he was studying the work of Raphael. Despite his disability Reynolds, a friend of the actor David Garrick and the celebrated lexicographer Dr Samuel Johnson, went on to become one of Britain's most distinguished artists, being knighted in 1769 and becoming official painter to the king. As happened with Beethoven and Goya, Reynolds's work as an artist changed with the onset of his deafness. The loss of hearing sharpened his way of seeing things and gave him clearer insights into his sitters. He did a self-portrait of himself with his hand cupped to his afflicted ear. He remained a fine speech-maker who impressed listeners with his erudition, although he did not like people using sign language, which he considered primitive.

Dr Johnson remained one of Reynolds's closest friends – largely because he, too, was hard of hearing. On one occasion, according to the latter's first biographer, James Boswell, Reynolds and Johnson went to the theatre together, but Johnson and, presumably, Reynolds could neither see nor hear. 'He [Johnson] was wrapped up in grave abstraction, and seemed quite a cloud amidst all the sunshine of glitter and gaiety.' Johnson spoke of deafness as 'one of the most desperate of human calamities'. His own hearing was so poor that he would routinely turn down invitations to attend social gatherings. Boswell lamented that his subject would not favour 'the ladies' with his company or attend 'parlour recitals' of music for the simple reason that he could not hear what was being said or played to him. On his deathbed, Boswell recalled, Johnson was less than charitable even to dignitaries of the Church who came to pray for him. 'Louder, my dear Sir,' he said to one of them, 'louder, I entreat you, or you pray in vain.'

Hearing loss came to the twentieth-century artist David Hockney in middle age. In 1993, a time when his work was extraordinarily popular and innovative, he wrote that it might appear to the casual onlooker that he was constantly surrounded by people. 'In fact,' he said, 'the only creatures close to me who are very warm are my dachshunds.' But Hockney found that his other senses, and especially his ways of seeing, became more acute. Hearing, he decided, was a spatial thing, and a person has to be located in space through sound as well as by sight. From this he moved on to the thought that, even though the human figure may be absent from much of his (post-1980) work, 'you can have the feeling of the human presence'. He added, 'What happens when artists use space with their imagination is an attempt to pull you, the spectator, in, to make you the figure in the picture.' He described his predicament in an idiosyncratic way. 'You are a lonely figure,' he wrote. 'Aren't we all? In the last few years, I have been lonely . . . Whereas before I might have enjoyed chatting away to people here and there,' he notes, 'I can't do it now.' One consequence has been that he now avoids, for instance, noisy restaurants and tends to avoid functions that are not intimate in character. He also emphasized the all-too-familiar isolating effect of hearing loss and said that he has stopped going to concerts and does not join in conversation in a crowded room.

The artist has strong views on hearing aids and particularly on the need to wear two at once. Paint them in bright colours and with great big knobs on, if you like, he says. 'So long as I can hear I don't mind.' Then, tellingly, he states, 'One simply reinvents oneself as a person with these plastic things stuck in your ears. Unless you are deaf, you have no idea what it is like.'

Two other artists, painting in totally different contexts, come to mind. One was Walter Geikie, who died in 1837 and who became deaf at the age of two. In his search for treatment and ways of communicating he spent some time as a senior pupil at the Edinburgh school of John Braidwood. Since Braidwood spent more time drinking than teaching, Geikie was often left in charge, before surrendering to his first love, which was drawing and sketching the people and buildings of Edinburgh. The drawings run into many hundreds and are nearly all characterized by the man's compassion and humour. The other artist, Vivian Pitchforth, was a Yorkshire watercolourist, who became deaf from shellfire in the last year of the First World War. Many of his works have a hypnotic stillness about them, almost as if he wanted to depict his deafness as well as the landscape in front of him. My wife and I have one, probably of the Yorkshire Dales, which we bought many years ago at a bargain price. I have always been struck by the absence of people and animals from the picture – its strange quietness!

In 1896, the year after the first performance of his play *The Importance of Being Earnest*, the playwright Oscar Wilde, whose father Sir William Wilde had been an eminent ear specialist, was in Wandsworth Prison, London. He had been sentenced for homosexuality offences, and while in the prison chapel he fell heavily, hitting his ear so that it bled. His mental and physical health deteriorated, and he was convinced that he was going mad. 'I am more like a great ape than ever,' he wrote to a friend following his release, continually in pain and without a penny to his name.

After an operation, which took place in a French hotel room and which Wilde described as 'most terrible' and a friend described as 'minor', he contracted meningitis and his hearing began to go. He thought frequently of death but urged his closest friends that when 'the trumpet of the Last Judgement' was sounded they should pretend they could not hear it. After his release from prison he had become a frequent visitor to the mortuary. Loss of hearing was almost certainly one of a number of final indignities he could not face.

The French writer Victor Hugo was not afraid of controversy in his lifetime and spent nearly twenty years of it living in exile in the Channel Islands. He lost his hearing towards the end of his life but, like Nelson Mandela, was able to find ways of coming to terms with it. One of his aphorisms has found its way into more than one work on hearing loss. 'What matters deafness of the ear', he asked, 'when the mind hears? The one true deafness, the incurable deafness, is that of the mind.' He was well into his eighties when he died in 1885.

W. Somerset Maugham, the British novelist and short-story writer, and before that a doctor at St Thomas's Hospital, London, was without hearing for the last ten years of his life. It did not staunch his flow of creativity, and in the late 1950s, when he won a literary prize, he spent the prize money on a new hearing aid – but only after he walked on to the beach near where he lived and thrown the old one into the sea.

A different sort of British writer, who is very much of the present, is Claire Rayner. She was born into what she calls 'real poverty' in the East End of London in 1931 and was a nurse and a midwife before she became a distinguished agony aunt, newspaper columnist and sometime novelist. It was my privilege not long ago to work with her when she was a contributor to a book of essays (called *Getting a Life*), which I edited for Help the Aged on aspects of what it meant to be old in Britain at the dawn of the twenty-first century.

Rayner's hearing loss was diagnosed when she was in her sixties. She insists that the news did not depress her, although she did admit that she was shy about it. Initially, she went through a phase of seeing the loss as 'a sign of decrepitude', but soon she realized it was important not to be reticent. Now, she makes no bones about her condition. 'I say, "I'm a bit deaf. Speak up."' She concedes that losing your hearing can affect your sense of identity and acknowledges that there are things that she sorely misses. 'I used to go to a lot of parties and hear lots of things I wasn't meant to hear. Now I can't hear adjoining conversations in restaurants ... I'm terrifically nosy, I find other people fascinating and miss out now on the gossipy bits. I have lost that pleasure.'

Clearly, however, she has not lost her disarming candour. 'I'm fine', she writes, 'in a tête-à-tête, but it's difficult in a crowded room, so I hold court and make people listen to me. I'm still getting as much fun out of life as I ever did. If you've got to live with something, you have to get on and do it.'

AND OTHERS

The evangelist Bramwell Booth, son of William Booth, founder of the Salvation Army, became deaf at the age of seventeen after spending too much time preaching in the open air when he had a heavy cold. He countered his hearing loss by using an ear trumpet and later, with mixed results, an electrically powered hearing aid. Salvation Army historians, who tend to report more with positive zeal than the objective truth sometimes warrants, say that 'by dint of patience and sympathy' he overcame his 'handicap' to such an extent that people talking with him scarcely noticed. His whole life, they added, was 'a conspicuous victory over deafness and the feeling of inferiority which deafness breeds'.

Among scientists the American inventor Thomas Edison stands out a mile. He was a person of prodigious energy and inventiveness and of wide-ranging interests who had become deaf at the age of twelve while working on a local railway. He has been credited with more than a thousand inventions, most famously his work on adapting the telephone and on producing the first electric light bulb. He, was, above all, a great rationalizer and improviser, communicating, when it suited him, by tapping on the knee, in a sort of Morse Code, of the person with whom he was talking. When at the theatre the woman he was to marry would tap out key words of the dialogue for him; he in turn proposed to her by tapping on her knee.

His rationalization was most apparent in his attitude to his own deafness. He thought it was an advantage in business transactions, since he demanded all key points in writing. He would bang on the table to get attention and squash the opposition, and thus win arguments. He said that his hearing impairment was not isolation but insulation and for relaxation would frequently go fishing but with no hook on the end of his line – so that the fish, like he himself, would not be disturbed. When asked at a party why he didn't invent some device that would improve his hearing he replied that he would then be quite unable to continue not hearing what he did not want to hear.

The list could go and on, providing insights and highlights from other people's lives, but I feel enough examples have been provided here to give some indication of how very different people have coped in their individual circumstances. There are, I know, many omissions: athletes, for example. There have been international footballers and cricketers, as well as sports people – Lester Piggott comes to mind – who have had hearing loss. In fact, a small encyclopaedia of biographies concentrating exclusively on people with hearing problems would be a substantial volume in its own right.

It will be noticed that a large number of those discussed in the lines above were deaf rather than hearing impaired, but this is partly because deafness is more total and more dramatic and eye-catching to write about, less private in a sense than the age-related hearing loss which is my main preoccupation. Perhaps another book will one day be written or collated bringing just these people's variegated experiences into a deservedly sharper focus.

SEVEN

Living with the loss

I T IS AN inescapable fact of any sensory loss, as it is of bereavement, that life carries on regardless for other people. The buses run as usual, just as they did yesterday and the day before, the chirpy chatter in the high street continues, although less audibly than before, and other ordinary things are still the main preoccupation of most people. Living with loss is not so much about adjustment as about retrogressive adjustment – getting back to where you were before the loss occurred. With a few exceptions, most individuals have their own preoccupations and, with the best will in the world, they don't really have the time or, often, the inclination to be bothered with yours. That's not paranoia. That's simply the way people are.

From its somewhat Olympian heights the British Medical Association tries to be helpful and does not beat about the bush. In late 2003 it was the co-publisher of a small pocket-sized book by Tony Wright called *Understanding Deafness and Tinnitus* and in doing so was offering a resource, which, the BMA said, doctors 'feel confident to recommend'. But to whom? We don't all have stiff upper lips, after all, and your average GP does not have a sideline in bookselling. True, the book is sometimes extraordinarily informative, but there were moments when its words could be at a highly technical level, which for the majority who remain scientifically untutored may have come across as perplexing rather than straightforwardly helpful: 'Electrocochleography (ECOG), brain-stem (BAEP), middle latency (MLEP) or cortical (CAEP) auditory evoked potentials all give different information about different parts of the auditory pathway,' it says on page 33. 'What is very important about this form of measurement technique is that the tester does not need the cooperation of the person to obtain a response.' What, I asked myself as I read, scratching my head vigorously, not even a heavy sigh?

Happily, however, page 1 is unambiguous in a different way and more to the point. Here the line between the clinical approach and the compassionate is, refreshingly, rather blurred. 'Becoming deaf, however severe the hearing loss, can be a miserable experience,' it says, by way of a minimal concession to human weakness. 'Unlike many other conditions, deafness is not immediately obvious to other people, and being unable to hear can cause many problems at work, at home and when socializing. People who have normal hearing frequently have little patience with those who do not hear so well. As it is often very difficult for deaf people to understand speech – which is perhaps the major characteristic that distinguishes us from other mammals – those who can hear give up trying to communicate with deaf people, get angry or just walk away.'

Small wonder, if the normally rational individual who is abandoned in this way is irrational in his or her reaction, and it is perhaps inevitable that hearing loss and deafness have been fertile areas for psychologists. Whether the consequential theories advanced by these psychologists have been fertile areas for the hearing impaired is open to question. Fashions, after all, change. One American psychologist, writing nearly fifty years ago, seems to belong to the ultra-simplistic, pull-yourself-together school of thinking. 'Why', asked Greydon Boyd, writing in a book published in 1959, 'is a hearing loss often associated with depression . . . ? It is probably a deep-seated fear of something threatening the individual which he does not understand.' The remedy, according to Boyd, seems to lie in being brutally tough with yourself. His thinking, I have been told, is dated and is seen as very much of his time, and psychology has moved on since he wrote. Even so, reading the words which now follow, my own reaction was one of anger and impatience and an unconscious (of course!) fantasy that the person who wrote them might rot in hell. 'The hearing-handicapped person', he declared, 'should mix with those with normal hearing and, above all, keep trying, as this course will lead to a better understanding of his own condition and ways of making the most of whatever hearing he has. Never should he use his handicap as a psychological crutch or an excuse for not attempting to accomplish things he ought to accomplish.'

A recourse to psychotherapy, not unreasonably, is suggested but so, too, is drug-induced twilight sleep or hypnosis on the basis that 'hearing may be restored by suggestion and giving the patient insight into the real cause of his deafness'. The patient had to understand that there was a direct relationship between the emotional disturbance and the physical disability. Who on earth, I wondered, was this man Boyd writing for? Am I alone in finding that last sentence faintly preposterous, more than a little incomprehensible or even irrelevant? One must hope that psychology, if only through the sophistication that is possible in psychotherapy, has moved on a little in the past half-century.

I do not know how many copies of Boyd's book were sold when it was published, but I suspect that Bill, Jim, Arthur, Michael and Bob, as well as Irene, Betty, Ivy, Tina, Erica and Carolyn, whom I meet every Wednesday morning at my lip-reading classes, would laugh like drains at hearing such advice. Teacher Jane, I am sure, would offer her conspiratorial smile and consign it to oblivion. What do you need, we asked ourselves one Wednesday morning, to learn lip-reading? Answers, in order of suggestion, were a willingness to engage in guesswork, light on the face of the teacher, a sense of humour, some knowledge of just what it is that is being talked about and not a little courage. If you think these needs hang rather uneasily together, remember that, for instance, to the less-than-experienced lip-reader 'GP' can look the same as 'chilblain' and that 'Scottish' looks like 'sausage'. Lip-reading is further discussed already.

However, in one area at least, the recalcitrant Boyd did sound a salutary warning. 'In desperation', he says, 'many people fall for quack medication and unnecessary operations. Other sufferers with nerve or middle-ear deafness and intact eardrums put pathetic faith in advertised ear-drops which cannot possibly help them.' I have dealt with such quackery in a Chapter 5.

It is an inescapable fact that living with almost any amount of deafness can be as arduous for the hearing as it is for the non-hearing. Both parties, especially if they live or work together, experience the loss, and both learn pretty quickly the truth enunciated in these three words: Hearing Damages Relationships. The strain on partnerships, and especially on hitherto close marital relationships, can be cruel. Conversation and everyday interaction which have hitherto been taken for granted become subject to an unfamiliar and unhealthy stress, which can occur at totally unpredictable moments and can lead to an unwonted sense of frustration, which in turn leads to resentment and grudge. Even between two hearing people a random failure to communicate can be a significant factor, if not *the* significant factor, when a relationship, including marriage, shows tell-tale signs of breaking down.

The impact of disability, including hearing loss, on marriage and the family has until recently barely been explored. However, the research organization Defeating Deafness has grasped this particular nettle and uncovered some disturbing facts in a recent survey, sponsored by Boots. One was that, although deafness was admitted to be taking a terrible toll on people's lives, they remained reluctant to seek help. 'Forty per cent of people questioned about the impact of hearing loss on their relationships said that communication with their partner had become more difficult. One in four said they now had to miss out on social events. However, on average it was six months before people sought medical help. Even worse, a third of those questioned waited more than two years before approaching their GP.'

When he became deaf, Jack Ashley was quick to point out that the business of helping deaf people, while a perfectly laudable exercise in itself, had to be carefully watched 'because it can so easily become patronizing'. Either that, he noted – in a refrain I have heard many times before and since – or people tend 'to equate loss of hearing with loss of reason'. Ashley was always resourceful and was fortunate in that he could draw upon reserves of his own resilience when they were most needed. He was also very fortunate, as he would be the first to admit, in having a loyal family around him. Reading the thoughts of his late wife Pauline, writing very eloquently on 'Deafness and the Family' (in a 1985 book of essays edited by Harold Orlans entitled *Adjustment to Hearing Loss*), it is immediately clear how much he came to depend on them. When the truth of her husband's deafness first became apparent, she noted darkly but realistically, the family knew that 'some harsh problems' would have to be faced, and when that truth became a reality, 'the doubts over Jack's job, and the happiness of the family, hung over us like a pall'. Like her husband, Pauline Ashley was a formidable person, and she was not afraid of underlining the downside of the impact of the loss on family life. 'The essential significance of deafness', she wrote, 'is that it takes away easy communication – and that is a two-way process. If the hearing and the deaf halves of a communicating team work together smoothly, the impact of deafness is lessened. But if the hearing half can't or won't join in, the communication falters or fails. Conversation is replaced by a monologue by the deaf person or, even worse, it dwindles away, leading to greater isolation for the deaf person.'

Generally, the hard-of-hearing individual develops his or her own methods of coping, just as anyone who lives or spends much time in that individual's company tries to do the same. The methods used are not always constructive and positive – there is, after all, no prescription – but, in their own terms, the individual concerned realizes soon enough that it is a matter of confronting the inevitable. Notionally at least, most such individuals do try their hardest – whatever their nearest and dearest might think – to somehow get used to the new darkness of their disability.

But too often it is other people who cannot get used to it. Take the case of Alison Hicking, an employment adviser for people with hearing loss in the East Midlands. Reading her newspaper on the train while commuting to work not long ago, she was startled when something was unexpectedly waved in her face. She looked up to see it was the ticket collector wanting to check her ticket. As she searched in her bag for it, the man began to make jokes about her ignoring him and started waving his hands around his ears before (jokingly) asking: 'Are you going deaf?' When Alison replied that she was indeed deaf, he went bright red, apologized and rushed off. By way of comment the RNID (which told the story in the December 2003 edition of its magazine *One in Seven*) noted, 'This kind of incident is far from rare. There are millions of deaf and hard-of-hearing people who face prejudice every day of their lives.'

Individuals with rather more insight than this ticket collector are prone to coming forward with the well-meaning suggestion that those with hearing loss should seek out others in a similar predicament, a common interest group. Easier said than done. In the London suburb where I live there is precisely such a group which meets every other Thursday lunch-time in the local scout hall. I am sure they are a very happy crowd and mutually supportive and positive in all sorts of ways, but with the best will in the world I found it hard not to hesitate when I looked at their agenda for the half-year when I contacted them. Two of the meetings, I noted, were devoted to talks – one on Bow Bells and the other on comic postcards. Four were allocated for games or other diversions – bingo, a game of putting, a quiz and other unspecified games – while two others were earmarked for parties and yet another for an 'entertainment' (from the person who had given the talk on comic postcards). These were hard-of-hearing events, I thought, that I would somehow have to do without, and I decided – with slight unease – to give the scout hall a miss.

But the human being, as well as being a notionally social animal, is also a functioning socio-economic entity. If, with hearing loss, you are of working age or of an age where you can still be useful and socially participate, then you may well spend less time smarting about what, for you, may be the shortcomings of events taking place at the scout hut and more time contemplating the often blatant discrimination that you now perceive in so many areas of human activity. During the summer of 2003, for instance, a substantial survey was carried out on small businesses, examining the changes they were planning to ensure equal access to their goods and services for deaf and hard-of-hearing customers. Two out of three of them were found to have made no plans, and only 2 per cent of the nearly four hundred businesses screened said they were planning to train staff in deaf awareness

Well-meaning people, by definition, tend to find ways of adapting how they will deal with you and talk to you; the less well-meaning ones will demonstrate a latent impatience and may even wish you were not there in the first place. They cannot necessarily be blamed for that; not being heard, for someone who has always thought that their way of speaking is perfectly understandable to everyone else, can be very irritating. But, as we've seen, Jack Ashley realized when he became deaf just who his real friends were. He also told how, when he was newly deaf and was accompanied to the hospital by his wife, who had her recently broken arm in a sling, it was his wife who got all the solicitude – even though he was the one who, on this occasion, had come for medical attention. Perhaps this could be called benign, or unconscious, discrimination.

There are some areas where the likely pitfalls can be charted and where the gentlest notions of political correctness may be applied. Students, for instance, who are intending to work with deaf people or individuals with hearing loss are given guidelines before they even start their studies. These guidelines bristle, as they should, with common-sense ways of signalling good intentions. The City Lit Centre for Deaf People in London, which runs courses for the well-intentioned, allowed me to attend, as an observer, one of its briefings. I heard some of the points to remember that would-be students would be advised to take on board before going into the field. Avoid the word 'help', it said, and use 'support' instead; avoid patronizing or talking down; do not be lenient; do not generalize; give the sort of treatment you would expect for yourself; encourage independence and confidence; be aware of different communication needs.

Such good intentions are all very well, of course, and it is comforting that they can be quantified and disseminated in appropriate settings. But there are some other areas where, lacking guidelines of any sort, you may find yourself practising your own discrimination with people you thought you knew well. Thus, you may find yourself thinking that individuals you have known for years seem to have started to misunderstand you more readily than they did previously. If you are also now misunderstanding or mis-hearing them, an intractable two-way tension occurs and new complications, which may devolve into something resembling an unsuspected intolerance or even discourtesy, may begin to take root. It is logical that, in this frame of mind, you may find there are social situations where it is difficult for you to participate and you may finish up speaking only when you are spoken to.

At the other extreme, a friend told me of visiting her elderly and hard-of-hearing father in a hospital ward – he was recovering from a stroke – and she had to almost shout everything she wanted to say to him. The whole ward, she reckoned, knew everything there was to know about the old man's finances by the time, half an hour or so later, that she had to go. Just as crowded places become no-go areas, there are some people, even people you thought you had known for many years, who become no-go people. And that goes for either side of the fence over which you are communicating.

Some features of the everyday environment take on a new and necessary significance. The postcard-sized logo incorporating a big ear, displayed in public buildings and enterprises, in theatres, shops and banks, catches your eye in a way it didn't before. This can only be a good thing because it probably means that an induction loop system has been installed on the premises and because it also unflinchingly reminds hearing folk that there are non-hearing folk among us. But, you may timidly think, it is not such a good thing, perhaps, because it draws attention to your new disability. The positive thing is that when it works – and it doesn't always, as several theatre managers faced with irate hard-of-hearing clients have been forced to admit – you can literally make yourself heard, and you can actually hear.

On the other hand, the logo can only be as effective as the people who control and use it. I was in my local branch of the National Westminster Bank the other day and couldn't hear what the counter clerk was saying from behind her security curtain of thick glass. I pointed out my hearing aid and then, somewhat beseechingly, gestured towards the well-meant logo of the ear, standing in its plastic holder on the counter. 'Oh that,' she said, very audibly, as she proceeded to take it off the counter and put it away in a drawer down below. We then proceeded to shout rather than talk our way through my ostensibly confidential business.

Invariably that logo is nowhere to be seen when you most need it, and the consequences of this can be disastrous. You go for a visit to your GP and you find, if you don't ask him or her to repeat themselves, that you are in fact guessing what they may be saying, which means, in turn, that you are very possibly giving the wrong, and therefore counter-productive, answers to their questions. Frustration is felt on all sides. The same frustration can arise in the hospital and in supermarkets and department stores and any number of crowded environments. Noisy shops, like railway stations and shopping centres, can be hell, as can trains and buses. I have long since given up all conversation, even on a one-to-one basis, while travelling on the London Underground.

Change is in the air for employers, their staff and their customers. The government's latest Disability Discrimination Act came into force in October 2004, and one of its strictures is that employers, even in small businesses, will have to pay greater attention to meeting the needs of disabled customers and staff. That will include the introduction of more flexible working hours and what government ministers sweetly describe as 'reasonable adjustments to the physical features of their premises'. This should help between 8 and 9 million people who represent potential over-the-counter sales of around £45 billion a year. This figure compares with the 250,000 calls a year that are coming in to the Disability Rights Commission from individuals and business people wanting to know the ramifications of the new Act.

Then there is the sensitive area of hearing loss and elementary justice. Tom Levitt, a Labour back-bencher, rhetorically asked the House of Commons not long ago how many magistrates use hearing aids. He didn't know, he said, but, given their age profile, probably more than most of us. How many courtrooms have installed loops to improve the quality of sound? Answer: Very few. 'It is not compulsory to fit them,' he added, 'but if they were, justice would at least be heard to be done.' It meant, in a nutshell, that the courts were generally failing to take account of the needs of literally millions of people in Britain today. The MP went on to quote from the thinking of the former chief inspector of prisons, the late Judge Stephen Tumim (who had two deaf children himself), who said: 'Magistrates tend to send more deaf people to prison on the basis that probation officers cannot deal with them adequately and I think the prisons make entirely inadequate arrangements.' To which Levitt himself added: 'Not only the court service is at fault. The police and the Prison Service, with some honourable exceptions, are equally guilty and, as far as I know [this was early 1999], so is the probation service . . . Some deaf prisoners do not understand how they got there, or why.'

An ability to hear and to exchange purposeful thoughts on what you hear is something that matters in court. The same thing applies to diplomatic receptions, events I used to attend regularly as a journalist (specializing as I did in foreign affairs) and to which I am still occasionally invited. But, because here it is the nuances of what is said as well as the words themselves that matter, they can throw up their own complications. The most potentially useful ones were invariably the most crowded, perhaps to honour a visiting VIP, and catching something from the exchanges between the hundreds of people in one room desperate to talk to one another could sometimes be essential.

On such occasions, even at the best of times and even with perfect hearing, audibility could be a serious problem. Without perfect hearing that serious problem becomes overwhelming. On one post-hearing-loss occasion I was invited with a few select others to the Czech Embassy for a round-table briefing being given by the country's then president Václav Havel. He was someone whom I had known off and on for several years and whose biography I had written some years before. Now, I found myself, not always successfully, straining every muscle to catch what he was saying. I knew that he always did speak in something of a monotone, but that didn't stop the feeling I suddenly had, in the company of somebody whom I had thought I knew reasonably well, that I was now on the outside looking in.

All sorts of specialists and advice-givers, like the brash psychologist quoted at the beginning of this chapter, counter these thoughts by saying that, as a hearing-impaired person, you should unashamedly stand up to be counted. Hearing loss is not your fault, they say, it is simply one of those problems that arise as you get older. Chirpily, they add that you shouldn't be shy about telling people you can't hear what they are saying, about telling them to speak up, to repeat themselves if need be, and don't omit, by the way, to ask them to stand not more than a few feet away from you and face the light so that you can try to read their lips. But if you are only a bit-part player in the conversation or if you are embarrassed as well as frustrated at your only partial ability to catch what is being said, the temptation not to bother and to opt out – and sometimes to feel inferior in some way – becomes enticingly strong. Anyway, it is not always easy to pass discreet suggestions to the most important person in the room or, in the case noted above, in the entire country.

One quasi-scientific complication is called selective deafness. It is, I note with a smile, something that affects hearing as well as non-hearing people. Every other day of the week, or so it sometimes seems, my wife suggests that I only hear what I want to hear and that I also deliberately switch off when I lose interest or the going gets rough. Certainly, one or both of us now seems able to grasp the wrong end of the stick after an exchange more frequently than we did in the old days. We like to think that we have a reasonably strong marriage, but it has to be acknowledged that clearing up misunderstandings has, inevitably, become a more laborious process than in the past. It is not surprising that the incidence of divorce is markedly higher than the average among couples where there is hearing loss. As I have already mentioned, my grandchildren, when they were small, quickly nicknamed me Grumpy Grandad when misunderstandings occurred between myself and them. Fortunately, the so-called grumpiness became something of a tired joke, but there are still situations where I have to join in, smiling blandly but without a real clue about what is actually going on. Even in the closest of circles deafness can be a joking matter.

It has been my intention throughout this book to be as honest as I could be. It has not always been a comfortable experience, but a great deal of anger, impatience and frustration – and some self-pity – has some-how had to be exorcized. But there have been other points of view to be taken into account, even some positive developments as a result of hear-ing loss. In a way that neither of us expected, my wife Angela has been a beneficiary and she was good enough to write down her views of how it has been to live with this process and how some things in our relation-ship have fundamentally changed. We first met in the early 1960s; her thoughts here relate to developments since the late 1990s:

Michael is not deaf, he tells me, but has hearing loss, a condition that became apparent over a period of some years. As a social worker I had encountered deaf people, but usually either children who were deaf or men or women who had become deaf suddenly through illness or trauma. Michael's mother was partially deaf as are several of his cousins, but they have been reluctant to admit to this disability and even to wear hearing aids.

I have learned now that there are many ways of covering up hearing loss, which Michael was adept at, so it was probably several years before I realized there was a problem. This happened suddenly one Christmas when members of the family were staying, and my sister-in-law, in her soft Irish voice, asked for 'a dish'. Michael repeated blankly 'A fish?' several times before she finally got the message across. 'Is he deaf?' she asked me quietly.

Often he did not hear the telephone or door bell, missing important contact with the outside world. However, once we realized there was a problem, we found remedies, helped of course by technology – a louder door bell and a louder telephone bell (free from British Telecom) and a portable telephone. Life immediately became easier to manage.

When you have lived with someone for a long time, you assume you know what they are going to say and don't always bother to listen properly. We were both guilty of this, and it has led on occasions to serious misunderstandings and even cross words. Not to be heard is difficult for most people, but not to be heard or understood by the most important person in your life is at the least irritating and, at the most, downright frustrating. A discussion about a play we had seen together at the National Theatre and Michael's mishearing of a key word led to a noisy row in the foyer. We had always used each other as sounding-boards on such occasions.

In the end Michael sought the help of professionals. There followed waiting lists, sometimes months in duration, for appointments and, eventually, a hearing test and a session with an audiologist. Hearing loss, a common complaint for older people, was obviously not a priority for the NHS. On getting the hearing aid, there were problems – such as when batteries ran out at crucial moments, or when he dropped 'the bloody thing' in a glass of water or even lost it. They all made life difficult for us both – but then we were rescued by moving house and another health authority.

Here he attended an audiology department which promptly provided an NHS hearing aid that actually worked. There was still background noise to contend with, but Michael was able to hear again. He now uses the aid religiously at all times, when there is a need to communicate – even in the middle of the night.

Two developments in the last few years have been significant in our adapting to Michael's hearing loss. First, he took early retirement. With hindsight, I have decided that one reason he did this may have been an unconscious, or even conscious, desire to escape from his life as a journalist where acute hearing is essential. Second, our roles changed. By unspoken agreement I now did much of the telephone communication, while Michael took over letters and the emails.

I had always considered Michael to be more extrovert than me, and I often left the task of communicating with other people to him. He speaks several languages, and on holidays abroad he did most of the interpreting. At parties, asking the way, making initial contacts, I had let Michael take the lead and it suited me. But this has gradually changed, and last year in France I had to use my rusty school French. This gave me confidence, but it was not easy for Michael as he had to stand by and watch me struggle in a role I was less familiar with.

In some areas, therefore, Michael has had to rely on me to a greater extent. This was a change for both of us, being highly independent individuals with lives and careers of our own. We were also thrown together more. Certain social situations are now avoided, such as eating in noisy restaurants, parties and large gatherings, and visits to the theatre are somewhat more difficult. Old friends, of course, have understood, but with new people it has not always been easy. But, for myself, I know that I have become more outgoing, confident and easy when talking to new people. I am also more alert in case I have to repeat a conversation or convey important information. There have been gains as well as losses.

In spite of irritations, tensions and some anger, we are finding ways of coping. But it is the casual, sometimes insignificant or even unheard remark that can be so important in the flow of conversation within a long-term relationship which has suffered. It means that when we are on car journeys we listen to the radio rather than talk to one another. But that, too, may have its advantages!

But, in spite of the foregoing, it cannot be stressed too often that hearing loss does not stop people from enjoying themselves. The hearing impaired can laugh as loudly and as often as the rest, when the words are clear and the mood takes them, even if it is a common matter of regret among those who are impaired that hearing loss means you may often miss the climactic words in a key sentence – something that is frequently delivered in a deliberately lowered voice. It can be disconcerting, even when you're feeling tough, when people in the group you are with suddenly burst out laughing and you haven't a clue why. You are reminded on such occasions that spontaneity is so often the meat in the sandwich of casual or social conversation and that to intervene with a plodding request to 'Please, say that again' can only destroy that spontaneity. It is another way of looking at cocktail-party deafness.

Places of entertainment have until now been slow in adapting their programmes to meet the needs of clientele with hearing loss. Two out of three of London's 'top attractions', according to an RNID survey carried out in early 2002, were not providing facilities for people with hearing problems. Museums, arts centres, theatres, cinemas and sports venues, said James Strachan – the then (hearing-impaired) Chief Executive of the RNID – were conducting their operations as if the several millions in the population with hearing problems simply did not exist. The Tower of London, the Planetarium and the National Portrait Gallery were all criticized, and it was noted that only 4 per cent of the city's theatres had captions, that very few cinemas provided subtitles for English-language films. Around two-thirds of the city's museums and art galleries provided no facilities on a consistent basis.

Six months later the charity's apparently tireless campaigners turned their sights on to television and subtitles and the estimated five million or so viewers who are obliged to make use of them – when they exist. Such subtitles were in fact first used in the early 1980s, but they were not an idea that caught on with any enthusiasm among the programme-makers. Since then some popular programmes, such as *Eastenders*, *Newsnight* and the World Cup, managed to provide them, but still the cry goes out from the articulate hearing impaired that they are missing out on their favourite viewing.

The campaign was adjudged by its organizers to have been a great success. More than 30,000 individuals were said to have sent postcards of protest to their Members of Parliament. One result was that the government of the time, with uncanny timing on the eve of a pending General Election, announced new legal minimum targets for subtitling on digital terrestrial channels. Four programmes out of every five had to have titles within ten years, compared with one out of every two at the time. ITV and Channel 5 had also to step up their service in this regard. Nor was that all. Under the Subtitles and Broadcasting Act of 2003 the BBC was committed to subtitle all of its programmes. Corresponding increases can be expected from the independent channels.

The subtitles that do appear are often of appalling quality, with letters missing, words misspelled – of no assistance, in other words, to a non-hearing person. But the good news is that the government is exerting pressure though its official watchdog, Ofcom, to set increasingly demanding targets for subtitling on new and existing television channels.

Hearing Concern also has its own monitoring groups that, on a regular basis, keep score of which channels are and which are not keeping in line with expectations and post the results on the internet. They and other campaigners remain determined to ensure that no quasi-legal loopholes are being exploited by the programme-makers. At the same time they are seeking higher standards. Some interested parties (who are not from Hearing Concern but who shall be nameless) with a knowledge of the art of subtitling said that the quality of television titles, at the beginning of 2004, had been deteriorating to a shocking extent. 'It was a highly topical programme with highly topical themes,' I was told in one instance, 'but I lost interest and switched the bloody thing off.'

Videos and video recorders are another vexed area. Most video recorders do not record teletext subtitles, but a separate teletext decoder can be used in harness. With DVDs there are a growing number of films available with subtitles, and the BBC has recently committed itself to including subtitles on all its own DVDs.

Hearing Concern has its own environmental aids committee, which devotes much attention to comfortable television viewing. A lot of us do it, after all. It also has its own list of devices and contraptions that are designed to increase both comfort and audibility but warns that they can be less than straightforward to set up. Do you mind, they recently asked members, being tethered to your set by a long lead? Do you want to be bothered with batteries? Do you need to wear a hearing aid all the time? Chastening reading, perhaps, but at least it's on a level that the ordinary listener or viewer might understand – that is, not too technical.

Cinema-going is now higher nationally than it has been for some thirty years but, until about the year 2000, it seemed that only foreign films and old films shown at film festivals for the deaf were the ones with subtitles. Now, as a result of even further lobbying and campaigning, this situation is beginning to change, and even some box-office hits are complying. But the campaigners remain, as campaigners should, dissatisfied. Would-be cinema-goers with hearing problems are being urged to write to (or email) their local cinema manager, underlining the gravity of their omission, while at the same time expressing heartfelt thanks in anticipation for the next subtitled screening!

At the latest count – towards the end of 2004 – about 130 of the 700 or so cinemas in Britain had taken into account the fact that the Disability Discrimination Act will apply to them and their hearing-impaired customers.

Many cinemas have drawn , where possible, on Film Council Funds to provide the latest digital subtitling equipment. At the start of the same year only 5 per cent of all cinemas had such equipment.

Meanwhile, the loop system is constantly being refined and developed. This is a system by which magnetic waves are sent out from a loop of wire attached to, for instance, a public-address system or a television set in your own sitting-room, which are responded to by what is known as a pick-up coil in the hearing aid. Larger loops are installed in some theatres, places of worship, concert halls, and so on. A cinema fitted with a loop or an infra-red system – to which most hearing aids can be harnessed – lets its potential audiences know that it is in place through newspaper advertisements, newsletters or notices pinned up in the foyer as you enter. Often there is a person on the cinema staff who has special responsibilities for the working of the system and the distribution of whatever ancillary equipment may be necessary. At the same time methods other than the loop are also being considered. One is to project the titles from a CD-Rom on to the screen. Another – cumbersome to use but apparently effective – is being developed in the USA and involves captions in mirror image at the back of the cinema, which are picked up by customers with their own individual reflecting panels and then superimposed on the screen, without, it is said, disturbing the person sitting next to you.

Some progress is also being made in the theatre. Stagetext, a charity set up a few years ago by a small group of men and women with hearing loss, is seeking to make captioning more viable and sophisticated where the complicated wiring of the loop system is not an option or where signing may not be possible. Peter Pullan, a former industrial chemist, is one of the small group, all hearing impaired, who run the charity. He waxes enthusiastic about the feedback from his audiences (from hearing and non-hearing individuals) and about future possibilities, which involve the use of a computer attached to a display unit near the stage. The current choice, he reckons, is between assisting at ten shows in ten theatres or one show in a hundred theatres. He opts, mainly for economic reasons, for the former. Meanwhile, based in Manchester, there is an organization called SPIT (Signed Performance in Theatre) that promotes the use of signed performances for the deaf with arts groups of all sorts in all parts of the country.

From an office inside the British Museum in London a team operating under the rather pertinent title, MAGIC (Museums and Galleries in the Capital) does what it can to facilitate the enjoyment of art, culture and history for all. It will help set up talks for specialist audiences and will cater, in the cultural sense, for family events, producing audiotexts or interpreted talks about specific displays. In the longer term, it would be nice if the C in MAGIC could be made to stand for the Country rather than Capital. Berwick-on-Tweed and Bodmin also have their share of the hard of hearing.

So much for leisure and culture. But what of the working environment? Here, too, it seems that comparatively little research has been done. However, some obvious conclusions have been reached and most notably that hearing-impaired people who work have a much harder time at their place of employment. There is a marked tendency among them to withdraw from bantering, or interacting at all, with work colleagues as there is for them to cease participating in social groups. At the same time, while some individuals with hearing loss may shrug their shoulders as if to say 'It's nothing', others may become more talkative and noisy, extrovert even, a means by which – according to psychologists – they do not have to concentrate on understanding what the other person may be saying. Still others attract attention by announcing that they have acquired aches and pains or some other condition – nothing to do with hearing loss – which they have not had before. This at least may evoke a measure of sympathy among those present, even if it is tempered by a smidgeon of scepticism.

Some research has been carried out on the impact of hearing loss on a person as it may be defined by examining their position at work. More than a third of the people in Britain who are deaf or hard of hearing are of working age. A pilot study carried out in early 2001 by Liz Daniel for Hearing Concern and other organizations looked at the workplace situation of a group of men with acquired hearing loss. She found that there appeared to be a general feeling among them that, while people did not actually lose their jobs, they did sense that 'their career path will be blocked and they might become stuck in dead-end jobs, with little or no perceived chance of moving on'.

This view has been endorsed by American researchers. They have found that employers were not keen to take on staff with hearing loss, on the grounds that communication on the shop floor and training might become difficult areas. In the late 1970s a British Society of Audiology researcher found that many people with hearing loss had had to change jobs, that their career opportunities were more difficult and that where they did have work they could well be underemployed. A survey in France in the early 1980s found that 50 per cent of deafened employees were sacked, while in Holland it was reported that hard-of-hearing employees finished up doing what they described as 'lonely' work.

Liz Daniel maintained that 'fear of rejection' was a big inhibiter at work as well as outside, stopping people from making new acquaintances and inducing a sense of isolation. The implication of this, she says, is that not hearing makes one less than a full, whole person, leading in turn to the view that the deaf or hard-of-hearing individual is 'ignorant, inferior and needs to be taken care of, an attitude of "they're not quite all there"'. This in turn led to the view that those who hear can dominate and indicate the only 'right way to communicate' and that anyway the hard of hearing should be able to 'cope'. Some hard-of-hearing workers said that, of course, they would have been willing to further their education through courses if they could, but this was 'impossible' or 'very difficult' now that they were hearing impaired.

The RNID has also carried out its own research in this area. In a report also published early in 2001 it was able to conclude that 'discrimination against deaf and hard-of-hearing people in the workplace is widespread', entailing a 'tragic' waste of human resources. Surveying more than four hundred companies and talking with more than a thousand deaf and hard-of-hearing individuals, its findings may be considered distinctly chastening. The tone of its report was mainly admonitory, although it did concede that many employers were worried about the cost of adjustments needed in the workplace to help an employee with hearing loss, even though statutory and other support was available.

Highlighting the government finding of a few months earlier that disabled people were twice as likely to be discriminated against than others when finding a job, the RNID paper agreed with the view that the chances of such people getting a job in the first place, and making the most of their skills if in work, were affected. Often discrimination arose as a result of 'fear, lack of awareness and inaction' on the part of the employers who did not realize that deaf or hard-of-hearing people were in fact capable of doing a good job. In other words, the disabled person had to come to terms with rejection as well as the disability. The silences of hearing loss, which I have discussed earlier, are compounded by the silences that rejection causes. Meanwhile, recent surveys of the salary levels of people with hearing loss have shown that 8 per cent of those working full time were earning less than the minimum wage, against just over 1 per cent in the national workforce as a whole.

The guidelines offered to would-be employers, like those that are offered to students, are based on humane common sense. They included: making the application process accessible, by asking applicants whether they required communication support at interview; asking, without making assumptions, deaf or hard-of-hearing peope what help they might need; providing deaf awareness training for hearing employees; providing a mentor or 'buddy' system where necessary.

Government legislation exists to help the deaf and hard of hearing get into work – even to the extent of paying for an interpreter or other 'human aid to communication' when you go for a job interview – and any employer with fifteen or more staff is required by law to make 'reasonable adjustments' to enable disabled people to work. Universities and colleges of further education tend, with some headline-making exceptions, to go out of their way to cater for deaf and hard-of-hearing students. But, as the RNID has trenchantly noted, 'most employers and deaf and hard-of-hearing people have never heard of [the government's] Access to Work scheme, let alone been helped by it'. Even in its own backyard, the government had problems: 'Government employment services', the RNID pointed out, 'are often inadequately equipped to communicate, with a serious shortage of professionals, such as sign-language interpreters, lip-speakers and speech-to-text operators.'

Clearly, discrimination and employment are areas of active concern for the RNID. It has established its own Employment, Training and Skills Service (ETSS) with offices strategically dotted about the country. Its staff work closely with local employment offices and give advice on what training needs might be required, on how to set about job searching and how to set about that crucial interview. Workshops, sometimes running for a few days, are held specifically for deaf and hard-of-hearing job-seekers. Once the applicant has found a job, the support continues, with a weather eye kept on the latest disability discrimination laws. In the small print the ETSS staff also concede that knock-backs do occur even in the best-regulated environments, and advice is, therefore, on hand to help rebuild battered confidence.

EIGHT

Grappling with the loss

ALL TOO OFTEN, it is a case of the dog that chases its own tail. The less you hear, the more vexed you become, which means that the more vexed you become, the less you are able to hear. Take the case of an older woman, not especially vexed but very sad, who wrote to me from Sidcup in Kent. 'All I ask', she said, 'is the chance before I depart this world to hold a conversation with my family and friends, in fact with everybody. To have to leave the company of my two lovely great-grandchildren because I cannot hear them is causing me deep depression. Where I once had a good sense of humour, etc., this now seems to be deserting me.'

You do not need a PhD to read the anguish that can come from such a situation. Even so, the bleak fact persists that, however many ingenious gadgets and remedies may be on offer, there are no cures for hearing loss and deafness. You have to fight for much of the time to survive. The same goes for an amputated limb: you can get a man-made replacement arm or leg, which may be versatile beyond imagining, but you cannot retrieve what is irrevocably lost. You can only replace it and make do with a sub-stitute.

Of course, as I have already noted, there are countless public per-sonalities as well as private individuals with hearing loss who have demonstrated a confidence to live normal lives. Nelson Mandela once told an interviewer that of course he didn't mind being questioned but warned that he would only be able to hear those questions he wanted to answer. His gregarious friend, former President Clinton, whose purchase of a hearing aid while in office sent sales rocketing in the USA remains as charismatic and in demand as ever. The extent to which these two and others like them may endure a very private anguish in less public situ-ations is anyone's guess.

Slowly but surely, and in spite of the reluctance of some well-placed organizations and public companies to engage in much-needed research, an awareness of hard-of-hearing people and their particular needs is increasing. A steady trickle of disability discrimination legislation has been passed, granting them new possibilities and, in some cases, enshrining new rights, notably in amendments to the Disability Discrimination Act; the health ministers in successive governments have endorsed and introduced measures to alleviate difficulties and hardships; and relentlessly vigorous campaigns, conducted by single-minded organizations concentrating on deafness and hearing loss, have seen some of their doggedly determined efforts achieve a measure of success. Even so, the disability-rights campaigners themselves, a number of whom are now resorting to unsubtle and direct action to achieve very reasonable objectives, remain sceptical. The official announcement that digital hearing aids should soon be available for all who need them is clearly a step in the right direction. But the reaction of those who spend their lives working with the hearing impaired is still tinged with scepticism. 'I'll believe that when I see it,' one of them told me.

Expertise, where it does exist, can be hard to access. My own experience in trying to reach the self-proclaimed source of expert knowledge in Britain about lip-reading, was limited but disheartening. I found the relevant university (in Manchester) and managed to track down the concerned department (Psychology and Speech Pathology), but no one was around that day. Admittedly it was July and the long summer vacation had begun, but there was not even someone available who could answer random queries. It will take about a fortnight, a department official said, so why not leave a message? So I did. After more than six months of waiting for them to phone me back I gave up the chase.

Then I tried to get through, on the internet, to the Association of Teachers of Lipreading to Adults (ATLA). I learned that they produce two issues a year of their trade magazine *Catchword*, but they wouldn't be able to send me one since they only make the publication available to ATLA members. I also learned that only qualified teachers could become members of ATLA. Unqualified teachers, however experienced and however skilled, are not suitable. Ordinary souls, according to the net, are not able to get even general information, not least because the association, based in Stoke-on-Trent, seems to have no resident office staff. The address is care of a Post Office box and there is no telephone number, only a fax. At least here was a context where the term 'dialogue of the deaf' might seem relevant – or at least appropriate.

On the ground, lip-reading itself is a less delicate area. It is, after all, something that most of us, hearing and non-hearing, do in certain circumstances. It is also a habit we acquire as part of growing up and which we perform without thinking about. But the formal version is something that Oliver Sacks, in his penetrating and memorable book *Seeing Voices*, has described as 'an extremely inadequate word for the complex art of observation, inference and inspired guesswork'. Some 75 per cent of lip-reading, he suggests, is a sort of inspired guessing or hypothesizing. Certainly, it is an art form which is only possible in the right environment, but some of us, say the experts, are not cut out for it and will never be able to do it.

If there are a lot of people around – say, at a party, in a restaurant, a reception, a theatre or a football ground – all of us have moments of watching the face, and especially the lips, of the person we want to hear. Some of us have developed fascinating ways of muddling through by, for instance, disguising the way we cup a hand behind a defective ear; others have honed the skills to an art form. I have been told by a police source of a totally deaf woman who assists the police by very successfully reading the lips of notional suspects who have been caught on closed circuit television cameras. For us more ordinary mortals, looking at lips is one thing, but the distractions of background noise can be such that even the most rudimentary lip-reading can be a matter of travelling hopefully through a series of exchanges without ever quite arriving. When the hearing aid you may be using also magnifies the background noise – often to a horrendous degree – and thus does nothing whatsoever to clarify the immediate conversation, the sense of helplessness is hard to avoid. Any suggestion of balance between what is heard and what is seen ceases to exist.

But, although lip-reading may seem an easy thing to practise, it is not. 'I read your lips,' was the slogan I saw recently on the T-shirt of a youth serving in a local coffee bar, 'but all I hear is blah blah blah . . .' Watching the lips of someone on television can be helpful when the sound is low but only when the person concerned speaks pure English, makes the approved lip movements, when you know the context of the words being spoken and when there is no distracting accent or speech impediment. It doesn't take very long to realize that the readable ones are rather in the minority. (While on the subject of television, hearing people may need reminding that if they are in the company of someone with hearing loss and the television is on, and they want to talk about what they have just heard or seen, they often needn't bother. The intrusive sounds coming from the box and a voice speaking even from a few feet away are not necessarily simultaneously manageable.)

One source of trouble arises from the fact that so many consonants, often among the first to go when hearing declines, look like each other on people's lips. Thus, 'mangle' and 'bungle' look the same on the lips – try saying them in front of the mirror – as do 'tortoise' and 'daughter', or 'cheat' and 'sheet', 'trick' and 'treat', 'London' and 'England', 'red' and 'green', or even 'passed' and 'pissed'. Other more guttural sounds, yielding phrases such as 'King Kong' or 'Good God', are difficult to discern and differentiate. And the negligible difference in the eye of the reader between, for instance, 'Come to tea on Saturday' and 'Come to dinner on Sunday' or between 'Life begins at forty' and 'Love begins at forty' can lead, theoretically anyway, to all sorts of complications. And whether 'life' or 'love' is available at 8.10, 9.10 or even 10.10 or at 3.15 or 3.50 is clearly something that should be clarified before you start preening yourself in expectation.

Such readings, even without any nuance, become almost impossible if the person speaking has a heavy moustache or face-smothering beard, or talks with his mouth full or hides his lips with his hand or a cigarette or a glass or a teacup. Lip-reading among the comparatively hairy Victorians must have been incomparably more difficult than it is in the early twenty-first century. It is surely no coincidence that the lip-reading classes which are run by the local authority tend nowadays to be taught by women or by clean-shaven men!

One of the advantages, the delights even, of these classes, in my suburban experience, is that they can be small and reassuring social get-togethers, discussing common problems and sharing ideas, under the skilled guidance of a teacher. All the participants at mine have become good friends as well as thoroughly competent fellow students. The class, which has been going for several years, has developed its own clearly defined codes of behaviour. One is that the men are actively encouraged to go off together at half-time for coffee or orange juice in the canteen below, taking turns, as in the pub, to pay for a round, while the women stay upstairs in the classroom to share their own intimacies over the contents of the vacuum flasks that each of them has brought with her. The only complication is that there is a very talkative class in the room next door which studies 'The Villages of Surrey'. They make a lot of noise when they have coffee and they seem to take a long time drinking it. The timing of our break varies accordingly.

From the exchanges in the classroom, it is clear that the class meets an important therapeutic need. Things are said which could be said in no other context about, for instance, the sense of loneliness, the consequences of misunderstanding what is or is not heard and the rage and the despair that intrude every so often in everyday life. There was laughter when Bill told of the occasion he saw his reflection in a shop window and realized with horror that he really had become an old man with a stick, 'just like one of those road signs which says "Beware, old people crossing"', and there was an uneasy silence when one of the women, aged fortysomething, told how at mealtimes with her husband and two daughters she was often silent and missed out because she couldn't hear what was being said and because the rest of the family momentarily forgot she could not hear.

But it is only when you start to practise lip-reading that the highly intricate mechanics of the operation in a social, as opposed to a learning, environment become apparent. If you are lucky in the person you are talking with, and once certain basic requirements are met, then progress seems very probable. Certainly some basic tips, or rules, have to be followed, which – be warned – if you are at a formal dinner or other organized do may be rather difficult to follow. It is advised, for instance:

> that you tell the person you are with that you do in fact lip-read before you start to talk

> that you seek out a quiet location in which to converse

that the person should stand or sit facing the light (if it is from behind, their face is in shadow)

that you sit or stand a few feet from each other

that you agree more or less on the subject of the exchange

that you don't feel embarrassed if you ask the person to repeat themselves

that, somehow or other, you keep an eye on the rest of the person's face as expressions can be just as expressive as the lips

that you have a pencil and a piece of paper at the ready just in case

that you stop the person speaking immediately you think you have missed something they may have said

One other tip that may not occur to you immediately, if the conversation has any intensity about it, is to remember that you should blink at regular intervals, especially if you wear contact lenses. It seems that to lip-read efficiently you have to be able to see clearly!

Then there is sign language, more frequently used by deaf people and comparatively rarely by those with age-related hearing loss. This is a procedure that has been used for centuries. It is thought to have been refined as a linguistic means of communication in medieval monasteries, where new-born deaf babies would be left on doorsteps to join the community, a community where the cowled teachers of the deaf would be constrained by hours of prayer or meditation or vows of silence. Some monks developed their own sign language for use at mealtimes.

Often individuals who are signing to each other may appear to non-signers to be shadow boxing or to be attempting their own sort of tick-tack messaging, as seen on the betting stands at race meetings. David Wright, in his wonderful book *Deafness*, first published in 1969, told how he saw 'arms whirl like windmills in a hurricane', a phenomenon he summarized as 'absolutely engrossing pandemonium'. But for those who have taken the trouble to learn it, it is an extraordinarily effective means of communication. The fact that it is also silent – apart from the odd gasp of astonishment or anger or amusement at what is being said – makes it intriguing, and oddly moving, to watch. Seeing half-a-dozen deaf people sitting around a table and animatedly signing with each other, some-times more than one at a time, with barely an audible sound being uttered, gives a rather daunting new meaning to assertiveness, but it can also be quite an uplifting experience.

There are between 50,000 and 70,000 users of British Sign Language as their first or preferred language in Britain today. The consensus among users is that much has been achieved through the use of BSL to improve many people's lives – and not just in their ability to communicate – and that still more will be gained with wider recognition and acceptability.

It is, of course, only one of a number of sign languages. Despite a known ability on the part of deaf people to understand one another, even across international frontiers, there are many different sign languages. Deaf children are known to develop, and quite quickly, their own impro-vised signs when they are together, although they soon discover that what they are doing is quite different from the formal BSL with which they may be confronted at a later stage. Meanwhile, BSL differs markedly from the sign language used in the USA, Ireland, China or any other country, including most countries in Europe. There are also regional dialects in sign language as in most spoken languages.

Sign language has had a long and chequered history, and it is a facility which has its opponents as well as its supporters and was one of the first and most contentious areas of feuding between some of the best-known US-based teachers of the deaf, Thomas and Edward Gallaudet on the one hand and Alexander Graham Bell on the other. Opposition, historically, came from the 'oralists' who wanted signing replaced by language and the use of proper words. The argument intensified to a point where it became a matter of controversy and was only resolved at Milan in 1880 when it was decided to ban signing, except in churches where priests could still use it for deaf congregations.

Today, most organizations associated with deafness and hearing loss are determined that sign language should again be respectable and that it should be as widely taught and used as possible. The RNID has its own CD-Rom and book of instruction, while the rather ponderously named Council for the Advancement of Communication with Deaf People, based at Durham University, claims to have all the course materials necessary, electronic and printed, for those wishing to take BSL examinations.

One of the beauties of sign language is that it can be used at functions where hearing, hard-of-hearing and deaf people are simultaneously present. Sign-language interpreters can tell deaf people what is being said, and lip-speakers can voicelessly repeat what a speaker has said so that they can be lip-read. For those who have no sign language, there are a very small number of highly skilled speech-to-text operators who type what is being said on to a phonetic keyboard which in turn reproduces, through a process called Palantype, what is being typed on to a television monitor or a large screen. Professional note-takers can be used where electronic facilities are not available, but where there are such facilities electronic note-taking enables a note-taker to type out the gist of a speaker's words that then appear on the deaf person's own screen.

Interestingly, interpreting along these lines is something that can be done on a totally confidential basis, and the interpreters themselves work to their own code of practice. The Communication Training Services arm of the RNID run specialist courses for interpreters likely to work in the vexed areas of job applications, police and court proceedings and health and social welfare proceedings. But, as individual Members of Parliament have recently indicated, very few policemen and publicly appointed social workers are fluent in the use of sign.

These are just some of the ways in which the individual can achieve communication at a personal level. At what might be called a more public level, where the majority of people participating are hearing, it is an entirely different proposition. In these places, taken as a whole, there is a wide gap between the art of the possible and what is practised. The sound barrier is not only a fact of deafness and hearing loss; it is also a factor in the attitudes, habits and laws of the society in which deaf and hard-of-hearing people also spend their lives.

NINE

Technology: an awesome overflow

TWO LIP-READING CLASSES, held in a classroom of a former grammar school, have joined forces for the afternoon. It is a nice break from routine, and from the undoubted strain of learning to lip-read, to allow for an introduction to technology. This means gadgets and contraptions, which the Americans usefully call assistive listening devices, or ALD, and what in Britain are more euphemistically known as environmental aids, things to make life more bearable – or is it accessible? – for people with hearing loss. Guidance on such things and their availability can be had in Britain from Hearing Concern, which travels to different parts of the country with an expert who dispenses wisdom from the back of an itinerant, and necessarily sponsored, converted minibus. But a minibus can only be in one place at a time. Today, some local authorities are doing roughly the same thing, on our terms!

We are to hear what little extras are available under local authority auspices to make life more comfortable for deaf and hard-of-hearing people. There are sixteen of us, average age over seventy, and we sit in three meek, expectant rows, classroom style, facing our well-lit teacher – as she has to be, according to the Good Practice Rules for Teachers of Lip-Reading! – and also the chart on which she normally writes up the key words with a heavy felt-tipped pen. A fresh blank sheet has been made available for our visitor. There is no soft, fitted carpet, as is demanded by the rules of this sort of encounter to muffle unwanted sounds, but the walls are plain and not garishly patterned, and therefore they will not be a distraction. We have pencils poised. I have chosen to sit near the front on this occasion for audibility reasons, but remember early school days as I do so and, succumbing for half a second to nostalgia, think for a moment of looking around to the back row where I used to sit to see if there are any familiar faces.

Since it is the twenty-first century, and since it is several decades since I left school, I content myself with showing to Bill, sitting on my right, a rather delectable quotation I had found the evening before while looking through that improbable little book *Deafness and Cheerfulness*. It is very relevant because it is a quotation about gadgetry but gadgetry from another age – even pre-dating Bill himself, now into his eighties. 'By the aid of a trumpet,' it said, 'one may listen longer with far less fatigue . . . Before I took it, others must make an effort to converse with me, which was often a source of deep regret . . . With the trumpet at my ear their labours were lessened and so my happiness promoted . . . Take a trumpet, fellow sufferer, by all means.' Bill chuckles, as I expected he would.

But then we are interrupted. At two o'clock on the dot Jo, who is a smartly dressed professional of thirtysomething, knocks and enters. She is from the local authority's Sensory Impairment Team, and she is carrying a heavy suitcase. She greets the teacher and mouths a carefully enunciated 'Hello' to everyone, smiling with her teeth at individuals she knows, presumably as clients. The class responds readily. There is even a slight buzz in the air. I begin to get the feeling that perhaps the technology ramifications of hearing loss are not so burdensome after all.

While Jo unloads her gear from a travel bag I read the little brochure that she has handed around as a preliminary accompaniment to her talk, a bit like handing around the order of service for some religious ritual. 'The Sensory Impairment Team', it says, 'is here to help anyone living in the borough whose hearing loss becomes a cause for concern. All our services are provided free of charge.' Sounds promising and a little bit incredible.

Her introductory words give some indication of the services and the pieces of equipment that can be obtained from the team – serving in this case in a mostly well-to-do London borough of almost 150,000. This statistic means that on this particular afternoon she is addressing approximately one ten thousandth of her potential clientele. Similar teams exist, she says, in most London boroughs, and anyone can contact them, from doctors and district nurses to any concerned individual. A team member will come to your own home to look at your problem and assist where possible, whether your hearing loss is severe or mild.

These service providers have managed to whittle down the more predictable and therefore manageable day-to-day hearing problems that confront the average hearing-loss household to less than a half a dozen: the telephone, the doorbell, the television, alarm clocks and smoke alarms. Phone bells and receivers can be modified to be louder (startlingly louder until you get used to them!) and can have flash units attached. So can front door bells which can, if you wish, have lights connected and deployed all over the house, which will light up when the door bell is rung or the telephone calls. Indeed, some door bells can be so loud as to frighten the innocent caller away. Then there are alarm clocks which you can place under your pillow so that they literally shake you awake at your required time. And there are smoke alarms which are liable to flash with a frightening vividness, breaking the boredom while you're trying to fry an egg.

In other words, these are devices which can alert you to an everyday sound you might miss, but there are also others that help, by enhancing the sound on radio or television or the telephone. Jo announces reassuringly that hearing television without disturbing whoever might be with you or your neighbours is a common area of difficulty. Loop systems can be set up, often entailing wires that trail around the room. The attached devices improve the sound of what you want to hear, but the wandering wires can be a danger to animals or small children.

Another sort of loop can enhance the television sound but in doing so gets in the way of normal conversation and even the front door bell and the telephone. Unfortunately, there seems to be no sort of loop which can cancel out the tiresome background music that so perversely accompanies so many television programmes, nor can it rectify the barely comprehensible dialect, accent or lack of clarity of your poorly spoken soap star. Finally, the loop can also be adapted for use in the car – poor communication between driver and co-driver is an area of notorious sensitivity in the hearing-loss world.

So much for the first steps in technology, which seem relatively straightforward. Jo closes the magic bag from which she has been extracting her samples and asks for questions. This part of the proceedings is not so straightforward. Almost immediately there is agitation and latent discontent in the air, an almost palpable sense of consumer dissatisfaction. In her answers Jo finds herself briskly acknowledging that indeed there are shortcomings in available services and over-the-counter equipment. In corroboration, as it were, one or two in the class come forward, saying they have tried using such things, including a much-talked-about throw-away hearing aid available from some high-street chemists. They don't express much consumer satisfaction, tending more to emphasize the limitations of such items from their personal experience. Even the much-vaunted digital hearing aid, Jo as conciliator emphasizes, is not the miracle that it is cracked up to be for everyone who tries one.

In her final peroration, and to murmurs of approval all around, she offers some general advice. 'Avoid at all costs the advertisements for "hearing solutions" that you may see in the newspaper. These have often been placed by salespeople and not by audiologists or manufacturers ... And remember, whatever equipment you get, whoever it's from, that your ear is constantly changing shape and capabilities ... But don't give up ... Be assured the technology is there – even the disturbance from background noise is being eliminated – but realistically, it will all take a long time to get through.'

A few days later I pay a visit to the modest offices of another local authority in another part of the country. I want to learn a little more about the sort of services that are usually available for the local deaf and hard-of-hearing people. I also inquire tentatively about the nature of the thinly veiled grievances that gnaw at the heart of worthy people like Jo who seek to keep the services going. What I hear does not, unfortunately, surprise me. Hearing problems, I am told – by a team leader of several years' experience – are increasingly being sidelined by the impact of the policies of the money-giving powers that be. In other words, the precise needs of an individual have to be carefully assessed and costed before the necessary money – always scarce – can be found to help.

Even the theoretically straightforward procedures for registering local people known to have hearing problems are becoming problematical. It is recognized that the number of such people is growing at an unprecedented rate – as statistical trends clearly show – and it is quietly conceded by officials that the hard-of-hearing category is tending as a result to be absorbed – or, as one person told me, dumped – more and more into the relatively amorphous older people's services category. The bright and sunny brave new world which we had glimpsed through the eyes of Auntie Jo was momentarily eclipsed. 'One consequence of this', I was told, by an angry and frustrated health worker, 'is that special little jobs, meeting very real needs, are, like special clients, getting lost.'

Later in the same week that Jo addressed us I found myself in a small basement meeting-room at the RNID, talking with a man who probably knows as much as anyone in Britain about the technology that is currently available to the deaf and hard of hearing. He is Brian Grover, and he has been with the organization for more than thirty years, almost all of his working life. He personally makes me a cup of instant coffee and proffers a saucer full of biscuits and then looks at my draft synopsis for this book, including a paragraph, which, I feel rather sheepishly, indicates my untutored perception of the technology situation. Noting a reference to the supposed organization and the possibilities of some sort of control in the appliance manufacturers' market, he says straight away: 'I certainly don't think there are any cartels at work among the manufacturers.'

One of the biggest problems for so many of the millions who are without hearing, says Grover, is the inaccessibility of the crucial information that is needed by those who could most readily use it. If you collect stamps, you can go to a stamp dealer and you can get specialist publications dealing with philately. If your eyesight needs rectifying, there are opticians and chemists. The RNID does its best. Its magazine *One in Seven* has a circulation of about 35,000, but even if three or four people read each copy it reaches only a tiny percentage of the millions directly concerned. It also has a magazine called *Solutions*, which is devoted to what is newly available in the technological marketplace.

The equipment which these magazines discuss and advertise, furthermore, which has usually passed through the hands of Brian and his monitoring team, is only some of what is available. This is because the RNID specialists tend to stay with what they know already to be good. 'But', Grover points out, 'there is the additional matter that there are no hearing equipment shops in the average high street the way there are opticians or even stamp collectors' shops.' Which is odd, he adds, because older people nowadays are often quite sophisticated consumers, and, what is more, they have more money in their wallets and purses than they used to have.

The inevitable consequence is that the equipment manufacturers' penetration of the market is depressingly lower than it could and should be. Hearing aids, being free on the NHS and not too difficult to get, are widely used – although nothing like as widely used as they could and should be – and the satisfaction level, or the newly acquired hearing capabilities, of those using them is around a more or less acceptable 70 per cent (90 per cent if they are digital). But the ancillary equipment, such as that described by Jo, tends – judging by sales or NHS take-up figures – to be less attractive to the potential consumer and is manufactured only by a declining number of specialist companies.

These tend to be bigger companies, some of them household names, because smaller companies cannot afford the research and development costs, and, often, the gadgets they send in to the specialist and concerned organizations for monitoring are non-starters. The RNID has a limited range of its own products but spends more time acting as consumer watchdog, through the columns of its house magazines and other carefully orchestrated publicity material. At one particularly sensitive moment in the conversation I manage to mishear Grover's message. 'At the RNID', I hear him say, 'we have the magazine and about thirty factories . . .' At which my ears prick up and I fleetingly revisit notions of a cartel and one which may be actually led by the RNID! Grover breaks into a big smile. 'No,' he says, calmly, to my raised eyebrow. 'I said thirty factsheets, not factories.'

The hearing aid is inevitably central to any study of how people deal with hearing loss. It has always been one of the ugliest contraptions known to man, but it has also become, in a relatively short period of time, the most convenient device and the one most used by the hearing impaired, 'amplifying speech sounds', as a text in front of me notes, 'so that they are audible but not uncomfortably loud'. Its history has been traced, in more than one publication, by the late Kenneth Berger, who has written that the first-known British patent was taken out in 1836, forty years before the telephone was invented by Alexander Graham Bell and fifty-six years before the first patent was granted, in the USA, for an aid that was electrically powered. An international hearing-aid association was formed in 1948, a year after the production of the first electronic 'master hearing aid' by a company called Beltone.

Hearing aids of ingenious but comparatively rudimentary design, bearing no resemblance whatsoever to the little things we now put in and around our ears, were being produced from about 1800. Some were quite extraordinarily elaborate, with one, which became known as the 'acoustic throne', catching the eye, and sometimes the ear, of the then chattering classes. It was a seat which had hollowed armrests carved into lions' heads. These hollows received sounds and fed them into a resonating box in the seat, which was in turn connected to a hearing tube. The public demand for such a seat does not seem to have been recorded – although acoustic easy chairs, as I mentioned earlier, became available in the 1900s.

Berger has also described what he calls 'bone conductors'. These were strips of wood or rods of metal, one end held between or touching the teeth of the person who was speaking while the other end was held in the same way by the person with hearing loss. This was adapted in due course so that one end of the rod had a semi-circular attachment which went around the throat of the speaker, while the other end was attached to the teeth or the forehead of the listener. Such devices, according to Berger, were 'quite effective but cumbersome'.

What was wanted, it soon became clear, was a device of real sophistication, one that would receive sound but which would also magnify it as it was transmitted. Here the breakthrough came in 1876 when Bell invented his telephone. If sounds could be carried over a distance, it was argued, could they not also be amplified for someone who could not hear? It was a question that intrigued Bell for many years but one that did not intrigue him as much as the telephone, to which he devoted most effort – in spite of the demands of a hearing-impaired partner and mother!

Berger's view was that the first experimental version of the first electric hearing aid may have been produced as early as 1895 by an American called Miller Reese Hutchison, better known subsequently for the invention of the klaxon. The same author is somewhat sceptical that the first hearing aid was produced in Vienna in 1900, adding that this particular item was of little use anyway if the speaker was much more than an arm's length away from the listener. It was one of Hutchison's aids that was used at her coronation by Queen Alexandra. Before long, however, the battery-powered carbon hearing aid had superseded this version.

The serious miniaturization of hearing aids took place after the Second World War. The Bell Telephone Company was still involved tangentially in the work and in late 1947 assembled the first transistor, which led to the production in the following year of the first hearing aid with a printed circuit and, four years later, to the first aid using a transistor as part of its equipment. The first all-transistor hearing aid, from a company called Microtone, became available in 1953. Ten years or so later came the first aid with an integrated circuit, with the first aid with an in-built directional microphone coming in 1969. By 1984, according to Berger, in-the-ear models were selling more than all other types of hearing aid combined.

During the course of 2003 the RNID conducted a survey to examine the relationship of people who are deaf or hard of hearing with the technology they use. It wanted to know what were the difficulties and challenges that came up in everyday lives. The aim was to obtain some guidance for the RNID's own technology researchers in charting their own development programmes.

The results may have surprised the dedicated researchers but will hardly have raised an eyebrow of the man or woman living in the average Hearing Loss Street. Almost nine out of every ten of the nearly 10,000 respondents, they found, were hearing-aid users. But of these only a very small proportion made frequent use of an induction loop, a wiring device which, used in conjunction with a T-setting on the hearing aid, is designed to give better quality to the sound you want to hear and to cut down on often tiresome background noise. The loop was synonymous with problems, respondents said, and they caused upset and annoyance. Ah, concluded the question-masters, that means more needs to be done to make loops more understandable and easier to use. Hardly the most startling conclusion.

Telephones, too, presented problems, although around a thousand of those replying were unable to use one at all. Thousands of others said the voice telephone was an 'upsetting' or 'annoying' piece of equipment, of whom around a thousand had difficulties making a call to friends or family. And what about applying some technology? Four out of every five replying said that they thought amplification and clearer sound would be helpful; more than one in three thought a built-in text display would help; and one in every two thought that a moving picture of the person you were talking to would help. The RNID replied, with perhaps a soupçon of self-satisfaction, that its technology directorate had these and related matters in hand.

Around 40 per cent of those replying to the questionnaire said that they used mobile telephones for voice calls, although 70 per cent of these said they had experienced 'annoying difficulties'. Almost a quarter, meanwhile, used mobiles for text messaging, of whom only 20 per cent experienced difficulties, often irritating or upsetting in character. These results may have bothered the RNID researchers, some of whom say that while some mobile telephones may give better reception and clearer sound they are not really suitable if you use a hearing aid.

The boffins at the RNID, as well as an unknown but relatively small number of others, perform a service of which any campaigning organization would be proud. Their work provides the basis of what the charity calls its 'Sound Advantage' service, which entails looking closely at gadgets and devices for the hard of hearing that are sent in to them by the manufacturers and passing on their adjudications and assessments, where appropriate, to the charity's publications and their readers. Commercially developed services, as well as goods, are investigated, and the result, according to RNID, is that each year more than 40,000 deaf and hard-of-hearing people benefit. Those who have doubts about a product purchased are routinely reassured they can send it back if they wish for a refund or exchange for a different product.

The latest catalogue, which lies on my desk as I write, runs to sixty-four pages and offers more than thirty items to help with ordinary listening; as many again to help with alerting (anything from a baby-alarm to a bed shaker to a vibrating wrist-watch); and more than forty items to help with telephones. Care packs are listed for use in hospitals, guest houses and hotels, and ear protection packs for those who experience discomfort during the take-off and landing of aircraft or who spend time in unacceptably noisy work or play environments. There is also something called aqua-ears to help you hear while swimming. It is an item, says the catalogue, stretching the reader's imagination, which is suitable for 'several uses', including allowing children to hear conversations while swimming underwater'.

TEN
Lights in the tunnel

A Victorian writer called Margaret Hungerford said that beauty was 'in the eye of the beholder'. The same could be said of the metaphorical tunnel in which some of us sometimes find ourselves in times of trouble. Entering one, so long as you are not claustrophobically inclined, can be an exciting experience. It was hard, the first time I went to France by a streamlined but otherwise quite ordinary railway train under the English Channel, not to feel a small quiver at the novelty of the experience. When I took my small grandchild on a boat along the dark and mysterious canals of an old lead mine under the Derbyshire hills he was thrilled to bits and very vocal. But not all tunnels evoke such positive responses.

Perceptions of the tunnel which the deaf or hearing-impaired person enters vary in intensity, just as the tunnel itself may vary in length. The nature of the tunnel depends, of course, on the experiences of the person concerned, but there can be no doubt that while you are in it it can seem to be tediously long and full of bends. Sometimes, as when a train breaks down in an actual tunnel or falters, you manage to endure the irksomeness while at the same time hoping that it will come to an end sooner rather than later. Sometimes it gets on top of you, and you begin to understand the anxiety, and even the panic, that may be endured by someone who hates confined spaces. And then, suddenly, there is a sense of relief as you realize that this tunnel really is coming to an end and you are reassured that there is about to be a refreshing burst of daylight.

John Ballantyne's father was, in John's words, a 'Man of the Cloth', a strong family man and deaf. On most occasions he was the sort of person who endured his tunnel, sustained by a mixture of faith and stoicism and taking in what he could through a rudimentary hearing aid which, as John now recalls, was at least the size of a large executive briefcase.

But sometimes even the stoicism cracked, and there were moments he simply could not take, as when the whole family sat down for a meal together. There were occasions when the minister would pick up his plate and go to eat alone in the kitchen. John somehow assimilated this experience and went on to become one of Britain's leading hearing specialists. Having retired professionally just a few years ago, he now insists, from his uniquely well-placed point of view, that, in addition to the changing social attitudes and developments, the combination of technological, medical and surgical advances mean that there is hope. There is daylight to come, and many personal tunnels will come to an end.

Interestingly, the same cautious optimism is conveyed by the UK Council on Deafness, which acts in the interest of more than eighty associated groups, many of them much bigger than itself, which are all actively concerned with aspects of deafness and hearing loss. Individuals working for the Council point to what they see as one of a number of symptomatic breakthroughs, the government's recent announcement that it has, at last, recognized as a separate language and was willing to fund the training of more teachers. 'Our members', one of the senior Council people said afterwards, 'are very positive at the moment. There is a lot going on.'

From the Council's vantage point, several metres, as it were, above ground level, that may appear to be the case. There is excitement, for example, in the fact that medical research has now reached the point where a new-born baby can be efficiently tested for hearing loss. But my older friends and relatives – the ones who are inclined bashfully, or ashamedly, to keep their hearing aids in their pocket or bedside drawer – are less excited: they have a very different perspective of the world.

The Council's stated aim is to influence policy-makers to achieve equality and rights for deaf and hearing-impaired people and to improve their quality of life. In addition to an eighty-strong membership, there are around 120 affiliates, including all shapes and sizes of voluntary organizations, public-sector bodies and private companies. 'Our diversity', says Jonathan Isaac, the Council's director, 'covers the full spectrum of deafness.'

Every few weeks, at a conference centre situated in an evocatively named thoroughfare, Britannia Street, not far from London's King Cross

Station, members and affiliates come together to express their feelings – often ones of anger and impatience – at government policy, or the lack of it, towards the deaf and hard of hearing. At one such gathering, which I attended in early March 2004, there was a heated debate concerning the barriers faced by deaf people when seeking access to the NHS. Several years before the RNID had noted that almost a quarter of deaf and hard-of-hearing people were walking out of their doctor's surgery unsure of what was wrong with them, while one in six said they would avoid going to the doctor's because there were too many communication problems for them to handle.

The RNID's latest report – mischievously titled *A Simple Cure* (published in the spring of 2004) – relates the experiences of nearly nine hundred deaf and hard-of-hearing people after visits to their GPs and to local hospitals, and it makes even starker reading. More than two out of every five responding, said the RNID, had told them they had found it difficult to communicate with NHS staff, and one in every three, a significant increase on the earlier figure, said they had left unclear about their condition. Seven out of every ten, who were reliant on sign language as their means of communication, said that the accident and emergency units to which they were admitted – in some instances after a journey of several hours – did not provide an interpreter. One deaf mother with a sick child told how 'it was only when I started crying that somebody came'.

The smaller-print situation was no better. Respondents told how nurses and even doctors shouted at them on the hospital ward when slow, measured speaking would have been acceptable and how several sets of pills had been handed over without clear (that is, audible) instructions as to what they were for. The disability discrimination laws were being broken, the RNID said, and approximately £20 million a year of NHS funds were being wasted – as well as benefits and other expenses incurred by the patients themselves.

A measure of deaf-awareness training, not just for consultants, doctors and nurses but also for desk receptionists – 'You have to get past them first,' said a voice from the floor – was what was required. Training seminars for such people should be instigated and notices posted at appropriate points announcing that hitherto inscrutable members of staff could, after all, communicate and/or that a loop system was in place. 'But how do you seriously complain when you are so vulnerable?' asked a delegate. To which Chris Underwood, RNID campaigns manager, pertinently replied: 'Too often, complaints are voiced only among friends or at the local deaf club. What about suggestions boxes at the GP's surgery or at the hospital?'

The requirement of the latest Disability Discrimination Act is that all NHS trusts, local boards and secondary-care groups should ensure that their services were fully accessible to disabled people. On being tackled by the RNID as to what she was going to do about such a dire situation, the responsible minister made the right noises. 'The Department of Health', she said, 'is committed to designing NHS service delivery around the needs of patients. It is for the service providers to implement the Disability Discrimination Act . . .' GPs' bodies said they were doing what they could to resolve the real problems arising, and the Royal College of Nursing said it was committed to effective disability and awareness training, etc., etc. We shall see.

Coming at a sensitive time in relation to the new disability legislation, the conference wasted no time in making sensitive points for all who cared to listen. Thus, a senior spokesman from Sign, the charity which studies and acts on the links between mental health and deafness, said that close to 3.5 million hearing-impaired people in Britain could be at risk from developing a mental health problem. Such a problem, he announced, could follow discrimination experienced by deaf people – such as a deaf woman who went to her GP complaining of stomach pains only to be fobbed off with a packet of antacids; within a few months she had died of cancer. What was needed, said Matthew James from Sign, was a deafness 'tsar', or ombudsman, appointed by the government to ensure that deafness was on the agenda of all government departments.

Even before the 2004 conference got under way there was no shortage of evidence that these barriers are in fact many and varied, as Anthony Cousins, a hard-of-hearing person, had recently found. His problem was an unwanted accumulation of wax in his hearing-aid ear, and writing in the quarterly magazine *Hearing Concern* he gave a detailed account of his efforts to deal with the problem. It began when his own doctor said that he should be referred to the local NHS hospital, and a letter should come with news of an appointment within two weeks. Three weeks later he heard from the hospital that the minimum waiting time for the removal of wax was twenty weeks.

In the interim the wax deposit had grown bigger and Cousins had become almost completely deaf. 'I tried', he wrote, 'to arrange an appointment at my surgery with another doctor but was refused. With the telephone barely audible I tried to get help. The Hearing Service Department told me: 'If you haven't got an NHS hearing aid, we cannot syringe.' NHS Direct told me, 'We only have nurses, no doctors and it needs a doctor's decision to syringe.' And the Accident and Emergency unit said, 'We haven't got the equipment here, so try NHS Direct.' The hospital's own ear, nose and throat department said: 'We don't see anyone without a referral letter.' The hapless Cousins finished calling, on a Sunday morning, at a private hospital near his home, where the ear was examined and found to be infected, and he was finally treated with a spray and a syringe. It cost him just under £200.

One among the total of around two hundred-odd members and affiliates of the UK Council is Britain's only charity dedicated to research into hearing loss, Defeating Deafness. It is based at the windswept, less-than-stylish end of London's Gray's Inn Road, two minutes' walk from the trade-union hall which was the venue for the conference just described. Its modest offices are small and cramped in a way that might have caught the imagination of Charles Dickens, who, by coincidence, had once lived less than a mile away. But the talk on the morning that I called was about the possibilities, not considered outrageous, that the charity could in fact be funding a British scientist in the field who might turn out to be a serious contender for the Nobel Prize for Physics.

A couple of decades ago, I am told, such a notion would have been dismissed with a raucous laugh as pointless and ridiculous. At that time precious little noteworthy research into hearing loss was going on in Britain, and what was in fact noteworthy was not being exploited vigorously enough by British industry. Much of the work that mattered was being done by academics and institutions in the USA and Australia. Now, the feeling is that British brains have woken up and are reasserting themselves and that original work that could be of real consequence is being undertaken in at least a handful of universities. On this corner of Britannia Street there is a feeling of momentum in the air; in these little offices there is a glimpse of some light in the tunnel.

Almost next door to Defeating Deafness a brave new world, costing around £10 million at 2004 prices and likely to have significant impact on the science and practicalities of deafness and hearing loss, is coming into being. This is University College London's spanking new Centre for Auditory Research, a project which brings under one roof, in purpose-built laboratories on three floors, several different strands of ongoing research that until now have been conducted by some of the best brains in the country in locations scattered about the country.

The project was originally proposed and has been planned, in meticulous detail, by a committee of nine UCL staff members. Situated as it is next to the Royal National Throat, Nose and Ear Hospital (RNTNEH) the theory is that there should be a capability to see the results of basic research applied in clinical practice. The main theme of the new centre, devoted to an area of theory and practice that has so often been dogged by controversy and disagreement, is collaboration. From some members of the committee of nine there are curious smiles when they talk of the politics of their calling, but there is general and solemn agreement that the role of the new centre should be to bury as many differences as possible in order to develop programmes 'to understand how the ear works and how it goes wrong'.

The new buildings will replace existing laboratories that, by common consent, have been very poorly housed at the Institute of Laryngology and Otology (ILO). In submitting their petition for funding, the committee was quite clear about what should be the new Centre's *raison d'être*. 'While technology is certain to advance in the next decade,' they said, 'progress in hearing science will, we believe, not keep pace with these developments unless facilities for very broadly based multi-disciplinary research are created . . . The research to be conducted in this centre will have a major impact on medicine.'

Individual members of the committee, blowing trumpets for their own ongoing research projects, are – not unexpectedly – unequivocal about the clamant need for new premises. Thus Professor Andrew Forge, billed as the principal applicant, states, 'The dilapidated state of my present laboratory space severely hampers proper exploitation of our research findings. We need to apply contemporary methodologies in cell and molecular biology, but the poor quality of the building fabric limits our ability to do so.' And, justifying the application, he and his committee pointed that some of the current research was going on in a converted run-down Victorian print works. They added that 'the ILO laboratories are dilapidated, inadequate and currently housed in scattered accommodation . . . They cannot be upgraded to the standard required for the foreseeable needs of the field.' It is in the context of this project that Defeating Deafness staff members have talked of the Nobel Prize quality of work now being done. The light at the end of the tunnel is not always an illusion.

As recently as the mid-1980s, just before Defeating Deafness came into being, the prognosis for the hearing-research profession was very different. Vivienne Michael, who came from a scientific research background herself to be the organization's chief executive, says that the haemorrhaging of the initiative away from Britain that had been occurring at that time – when British research had previously been a leader in key fields – was devastating. The country found that it had no culture for research because research itself was not seen as a priority in concerned organizations and big companies when it came to funding, and, besides, deafness and hearing loss were not in the least glamorous. Michael talks of implicit anomalies in the comparatively recent proliferation of organizations which are now concerned with aspects of deafness and hearing loss, something which has led to a situation where the overriding cause has become beset by its own divisions. Each organization has found itself trespassing on the one next door, and all have been competing for the few funds available.

However, the fact is that Defeating Deafness did emerge in 1985 and, apart from inevitable setbacks caused by intermittent blockages in the flow of voluntary funds, it has been a pioneering force ever since. It has facilitated a number of what it calls 'important scientific breakthroughs', including the development of new technologies for screening babies for deafness, for new therapies to relieve tinnitus and for the design and production of more effective hearing aids and cochlear implants. The ultimate aim, it corporately declares, is to find cures for disabilities that are recognized to be neglected as well as distressing.

Good intentions, it has since transpired, have not been enough, and the old divisions of the controversy-laden world of the deaf and those who seek to work with them soon surfaced. When Defeating Deafness ploughed funds for research, initially using newts and birds, into the possibility and then into the reality of cochlear implants for children, the hate mail started to arrive because there was an unfounded suspicion that children were being used for clinical research. Vivienne Michael, with a very brittle smile, recalls that she received letters in which she was compared with the Nazis and informed that her funding was allegedly going into methods that had more to do with the 'research' methods of the concentration camp than the niceties of better hearing. But that storm, for the moment, has passed, and the cochlear implant even for small children, although still controversial, is less a subject for heated debate than it was. (Some specialists say using the implant with small children is in fact the best way of using it.) The work, in this and other areas, continues.

One of these other areas is age-related hearing loss, where Defeating Deafness has been pleased to pat itself on the back with the pronouncement that 'it is only a matter of time' – perhaps five to seven years – before therapies to prevent the deterioration of hearing or medical treatments for it become available. It has funded research to identify chemical agents and genes which might prevent hair cell death or which might trigger their regeneration. It has looked closely into the links between exposure to loud noise, whether at work or at leisure, and hearing loss, and, alongside a number of other organizations, it has looked into ways of improving what is seen to be still very elementary technology. With a grant from one of the larger clearing banks it is also examining what linkage there may be between defective hearing and Alzheimer's disease.

Noise-induced hearing loss is a research area in its own right. But what legally constitutes an unsafe noise level has yet to be determined, and the official advice for the time being is that breaks of, say, ten minutes or quarter of an hour every hour should be taken where the hearer thinks what he or she is hearing is excessive. One estimate is that more than a million people in Britain are exposed to damaging noise levels and close to 200,000 have hearing problems from the same cause.

Some regulations, including those specifically directed at noise at work, enacted in 1989, are being monitored in Britain by the Health and

Safety Executive, and as I write they are in the process of being honed to comply with relevant European Union directives. A regularly updated pack, advising on how to monitor noise and its regulation and covering the duties of employers, is available from the HSE offices in Sheffield. But Defeating Deafness has meanwhile pointed out that employers are obliged to take steps to protect the hearing of their workforce. Information, for instance, should be given on how employees can protect their ears; ear-protection zones should be signposted; and ear muffs should be made available where required, along with instructions on how to use them effectively. How the shop-floor worker is able to ensure that such measures are taken can be a complicated affair and, clearly, can depend on what sort of boss is in charge. If you can't hear what a person is saying to you from three feet away there is considerable cause for concern; if you can't hear them at six feet you should beware.

Defeating Deafness says it has given a great deal of financial support to research in this area but that much more remains to be done. There is some excitement that a drug is emerging which can cut noise-induced damage by as much as 50 per cent, but clinical trials, which cost money, are still needed. In addition it has had teams looking at new treatments for tinnitus, acquired as a result of undue noise, and at the damage to tiny hair cells in the ear caused specifically by noise.

Hearing loss in small children is also being researched. While, in general, the toys in the shops are manufactured, as far as their noise output is concerned, within specific guidelines and according to stipulated British Standards, some questionable ones do still get through the net. For this reason, so-called talking toys, according to researchers working with Defeating Deafness, should be treated with a degree of circumspection. Some musical roundabouts, toy aeroplanes and fire engines can be very noisy indeed; rattles and drum kits can be even noisier. Problems can arise if the child likes to hold new toys close to the ear, and the researchers' suggestion is that prospective buyers should listen to the toy themselves before buying. If the child is known to have sensitive or vulnerable hearing, then the use of ear plugs should be encouraged. Heavily pregnant women are, meanwhile, reminded that excessive noise can carry risks for the unborn child.

In the heady commercial world and away from the research laboratories, and in a proclaimed endeavour to make available some of the fruits of research, Boots the Chemist introduced a string of its own across-the-counter hearing centres at a selected number of its high-street branches some years ago. It did so under the label Boots Hearingcare and touted for custom on the premise that looking after your hearing should be as easy as looking after your eyesight, and, indeed, the operation was billed in the accounts as part of Boots Opticians Ltd. From the hearing-impaired consumers' point of view it could only be a step in the right direction. Then in the autumn of 2003 this particular operation was bought out by the main provider involved. This was David Ormerod Hearing Centres, based in Llandudno, North Wales, which, with a faint touch of grandiloquence, now calls itself David Ormerod Hearing Centres at Boots. What had started as a one-man business in the Merseyside town of Birkenhead in the early 1960s now operates more than a hundred centres country-wide. These are not only in Boots and other stores but also in doctor's practices and, in partnership, in some NHS hospitals. It is not only approved by the Hearing Aid Council, its managing director – Peter Ormerod, son of the founder – actually sits on key committees of that Council. As the incidence of hearing loss increases, in proportion with the growing number of people living longer, so the future, according to Peter Ormerod, is getting brighter.

As he hands over details of free helplines and home visits, of rehabilitation programmes and money-back guarantees, Ormerod emphasizes that he is very satisfied that technological developments are on his side. Although a dispenser and not a manufacturer he is pleased enough to see the beginning of the end of analogue devices, including hearing aids, and the increasing trends towards digitalization. He is also pleased to note that, in his view anyway, it is increasingly acceptable to be seen 'wearing something in your ear'. He seems to be well satisfied with the way hearing-equipment services are going, and what he says indicates very clearly that the lines that until now have separated the options of going to your GP, at no charge, and going private, for the price of a good pair of spectacles, are getting more and more blurred. Policy-making, in the corridors of the NHS and elsewhere, will clearly have some interesting conundrums to deal with in the years ahead.

Defeating Deafness has carried out its own (sponsored) research into the attitudes that people have to hearing loss. Some disturbing facts came to light. One was that, although deafness was admitted to be taking a terrible toll on people's lives, they remained reluctant to seek help. 'Deafness damages relationships,' the organization warned. 'Forty per cent of people questioned about the impact of hearing loss on their relationships said that communication with their partner had become more difficult. One in four said they now had to miss out on social events. However, on average it was six months before people sought medical help. Even worse, a third of those questioned waited more than two years before approaching their GP.'

There has also been interesting research by the same organization into individual relationships with hearing aids, before and after they have been acquired. In a couple of pithy sentences they convey a wide range of deep feelings. 'The stigma attached to deafness', it noted, 'prevents many seeking help and advice about hearing aids. Even when hearing aids are prescribed, the poor performance of many aids deters people from using them.'

In another part of London, Hammersmith, are the refreshingly open-plan offices of Hearing Concern. This is another small but quietly effective charity which is dedicated, according to its mission statement, to improving the quality of life for those who are hard of hearing. Its chief executive is Fiona Robertson, who, like John Ballantyne's father, is a strong-minded Scot. On limited financial resources – something borne with a very Scottish stoicism – it also seeks, through a variety of means, to raise public and professional awareness of the issues associated with hearing loss. Where to draw a line around activities as potentially vast as that is not something discussed, but the inability actually to define the task in hand has done nothing to diminish enthusiasm.

The organization started soon after the end of the Second World War as the British Association of the Hard of Hearing. Then, individuals who had suffered on the front line and women who had suffered in munitions factories and other noisy places on the home front came together in their hard-of-hearing clubs and decided to amalgamate some of their resources in the common cause. The greatest need at the time was some sort of social life and also to convince hearing people that those with hearing loss were not to be treated with indifference or derision. The need still governs the organization's policies and thinking. The result is that today its minuscule staff has the backing of an estimated five thousand members and volunteers in all parts of the country, campaigning on a variety of perennially significant issues. Hard-of-hearing clubs had started after the First World War, the first ones being formed in Edinburgh and Glasgow, with others following in the industrial north of England and, later, the south of England as well.

Fiona Robertson is a former nurse who is hearing impaired herself. She talks openly of the need to reach out to millions of people who are continuing to experience difficulties as a result of hearing loss or who are reluctant to seek help. They are not so reluctant on the telephone, apparently, and Hearing Concern's helpline is one of its busiest services. The key words governing the organization's work seem to be 'awareness', 'access', 'information', 'advice' and 'support', which seems straightforward enough. But the calling has its difficult moments: the Hearing Concern mobile advisory service bus, which carries the message and answers queries in all parts of the Home Counties, has been known to stand for four hours (in one well-heeled suburb) and get no visitors at all. A 'toughening' experience, says Tim Partridge, the Welshman in charge.

The exclusion (Hearing Concern's word) of deaf and hard-of-hearing people from digital television, radio and telephone services has been a major preoccupation, and there has been a measurable impact on legislation. Concessions have also been won for diploma nursing students with hearing problems who, as a result of intense lobbying, have become eligible for disabled students' allowances. Meanwhile, it must have been galling to report that the organization's Sympathetic Hearing Scheme, which sought to educate the wider public in the needs of hearing-impaired people, had to be – temporarily? – suspended for lack of funds.

The Link Centre for Deafened People, based in Eastbourne, seems like a cross between an old-fashioned and highly efficient social-work department and an old-fashioned and caring business school. It was established just over thirty years ago as a charity, governed by a trust – with several deafened people serving as trustees – and says that it is the only national organization in the UK working exclusively with deafened adults, their families and the deafened professionals supporting them. It has just under twenty permanent members of staff and almost as many tutor/trainers and more than seventy highy trained and fully supported volunteers.

Its target clientele are the 125,000 or so deafened adults in Britain, people who grew up hearing and then became profoundly deaf after their mid-teens – not really the subject of this book. But the work that Link does, and the measured maturity of approach that seems to characterize that work, suggests a sophistication of method that other organizations dealing with the hearing impaired would do well to copy. Many individuals with hearing loss, who outnumber Link's clientele by about sixty or seventy to one, would surely benefit from a Link type of treatment. Aware of this fact, no doubt, Link is engaged with a university in London in a three-year research study on the impact of hearing loss in older people and their families. Link's chief executive, Dr Lorraine Gailey, has conceded there is what she calls 'a severe lack of resources' as well as inadequate skills and knowledge about the needs of such people.

The organization has accumulated a vast amount of specialist knowledge and expertise in its chosen area over the last thirty years, but its supporters admit it still has a long way to go. John Graham, one of the country's top ear, nose and throat specialists, wants to see more psychological therapy available for deafened people and is convinced that there will be big developments over the next decade. Even health professionals have tended to misunderstand and overlook the needs of such people. 'Each one of them', he has said, 'needs strategies for dealing with emotional and communication hurdles.'

Meanwhile, throughout the year Link continues to run its workshops and study days to train anyone who works with deafened adults, from audiologists and psychologists to lip-reading teachers and social workers. It runs workshops and small therapeutic social support groups, often bringing one family where there is a deafened person together with another in the same boat. Afterwards, contact is maintained with the client for a set period and assessments are sent to his or her GP, hospital consultant and other relevant agencies. 'Who comes?' Link asks rhetorically in one of its leaflets, and its answer: 'People just like you, really.' But not yet, apparently, men and women with age-related hearing loss.

The question of rehabilitation for the hearing impaired was raised with me as I was researching this book in a letter I received from a woman in Edinburgh called Sarah Kilbey. She has been wearing hearing aids for around forty years – since her teens – and said she felt strongly about the whole question of the lack of rehabilitation for people affected by hearing loss. 'On being fitted with a new aid, patients get ten to twenty minutes at most and are then told to go away and live with it. But hearing aids take *months* to get used to. There are so many component parts, and so many different situations in which they have to be managed . . . I am also appalled at the ignorance and lack of knowledge about what equipment and help is available on the part of professionals like doctors and health visitors.' And so on – after no less than forty years of first-hand experience.

Ms Kilbey's sentiments were echoed by a man called Bob Green who wrote to me from Bristol. He argued that the deeply felt sentiments of impatience that I had expressed about hearing loss in the article I wrote for the *Guardian* should be given to all new hearing-aid users and then passed on to 'friends, family, lovers and work mates'. Ruth Pilkington, writing from the island of Jersey, announced that she would pass on my piece to members of her family – 'probably the worst offenders in the deaf-awareness stakes'.

Ten years younger than Link is an organization based at Saunderton in Buckinghamshire, with offshoots in North Yorkshire and Oxfordshire, called simply Hearing Dogs for Deaf People. All of its work, it says, as do so many organizations associated with deafness and hearing loss, has to rely on the generosity of the public. Publicity material offering anecdotal evidence of the efficacy of its work also carries a form you can fill in, offering anything from fifty pence, which helps to feed a puppy-in-training for one day, to £5000, which would make you an exclusive sponsor of a hearing dog's training to act as 'assistant and companion' – and *de facto* friend for life – for individuals who are severely or profoundly deaf.

The dogs, which are usually unwanted strays or acquired from dogs' homes such as Battersea, perform remarkable feats. They are trained to alert their owners to all significant sounds (including door bells and telephones), to get them up in the morning and go everywhere with them as watchful eyes-and-ears companions, but the consensus judgement of their owners seems to be that they have very decided characters in their own right. The animals come to their owners free of charge, and the organization says that more than half-a-million people in Britain have severe or profound hearing loss and could benefit from using them. Given the loneliness endured by several times that number of pensioners with ordinary hearing loss, perhaps they could benefit, too.

But there are not enough dogs for everyone. For the millions who are deaf or who have hearing loss it is an increase in deaf awareness that would, in many cases, do as much as even the most affectionate dog to assist them in meeting the deficits of their condition. Hearing loss is, in most cases, more than anything else a private matter. Those affected want social interaction as much, or as little, as anyone else – but they have invisible difficulties in interacting at an efficient level. A dog can obviously help and can even be a charming sort of bridge between a hearing-impaired owner and a hearing person, but the persisting difficulties remain.

It will soon be forty years since the newly deafened Jack Ashley decided, after some hesitation, to take the plunge and, in a public meeting, give voice to his anger at public attitudes to deaf people and the discrimination that these attitudes fostered. He did so by underlining the fact that there was at the time no proper provision for rehabilitation centres or for training lip-reading teachers and declared that, 'If the blind were deprived of sticks and guide dogs, or the crippled denied crutches, there would be an outcry' – to which one can only add, with a sigh, 'Hear, hear!' More than a generation on and there is still scope for the same justifiable anger.

Hearing therapists, who are currently very thin on the ground, could have a key role to play. At the moment it is a matter of locating the nearest therapist to you through the audiology department of your local hospital, booking an appointment and then waiting. They exist to provide what, in the jargon of the moment, is called 'a comprehensive rehabilitation service', dispensing information, advice and, where appropriate, counselling to people with hearing difficulties. The discipline of hearing therapy is one which is being enhanced at the moment, with more recognition being given to formal training at university level and the qualifications needed to practise. An increasing, if tiny, number of graduates are applying.

As I write, there are far fewer than two hundred of them practising in the whole of Britain, which works out at one therapist for every 60,000 notional clients. In my limited experience, nobody who is deaf or hard of hearing wants to be spoon-fed with counselling or advice. But a knowledgeable ear from an increased number of sympathetic specialists to hear their qualms, in the wake of some really satisfactory treatment, efficiently given, from the medical profession and those who work with it, would save a lot of time, money and anguish. It would also change a great many lives.

And it would also, I submit, be a civilized way of eliminating some of the grumpiness in suburbia and elsewhere. Almost no one since Charles Dickens's Scrooge would say out loud that they enjoy being grumpy, and even Scrooge in the end relented. This was because the barriers that he had perceived as standing between him and the non-grumpy world had been broken down and he no longer felt he was an ostracized stranger among his fellow humans. There are, I know from personal experience, a lot of people with hearing loss out there – distant relatives of Scrooge perhaps – who feel there are an untold number of different barriers, however invisible, between themselves and the hearing world, and they would give a great deal for those barriers to be broken down.

After all, they never asked for them to be erected in the first place.

SELECT BIBLIOGRAPHY

Ashley, Jack, *Acts of Defiance*, London: Reinhardt, 1992

— *Journey into Silence*, London: Bodley Head, 1973

Boyd, Greydon, *Hearing Loss: What Can Be Done About It*, New York and
    Philadelphia: Lippincott, 1959

Branson, Jan and Don Miller, *Damned for Their Difference: The Cultural Construction of
    Deaf People as Disabled*, Washington, DC: Gallaudet University Press, 2002

Coni, N., W. Davison and S. Webster, *Ageing: The Facts*, Oxford: Oxford University
    Press, 1992

Freeland, Andrew, *Deafness: The Facts*, Oxford: Oxford University Press, 1989

Glennie, Evelyn, *Good Vibrations: My Autobiography*, London: Century Hutchinson,
    1990

Graham, John and Mike Martin (eds), *Ballantyne's Deafness*, London: Whurr
    Publishing (6th edn), 2001

Hale, Sheila, *The Man Who Lost His Language*, London: Allen Lane, 2002

Hall, Michael with Simon Rattle, *Leaving Home*, London: Faber and Faber, 1996

Harvey, Michael, 'What's On Your Mind?', *Hearing Loss Magazine*, January 2004

Hockney, David, *That's the Way I See It*, Nikos Stangos (ed.), London: Thames and
    Hudson, 1993

Holiday, Kate, 'Goodbye Silence', *Hearing Therapy*, Winter 2002

Jackson, A.W., *Deafness and Cheerfulness*, Boston: Little Brown, 1902

Jones, Lesley, Jim Kyle and Peter Wood (eds), *Words Apart: Losing Your Hearing as an
    Adult*, London: Tavistock Publications, 1987

Kureishi, Hanif, 'Loose Tongues and Liberty', *Guardian*, 7 June 2003

Lane, Harlan, *The Mask of Benevolence: Disabling the Deaf Community*, New York:
    Alfred A. Knopf, 1992

— *When the Mind Hears: A History of the Deaf*, New York: Random House, 1984

Lewycka, Marina, *Caring for Someone with a Hearing Loss*, London: Age Concern
    Books, 2001

Martin, Michael and Brian Grover, *Ears and Hearing*, London: Macdonald Optima, 1990

Mirzoeff, Nicholas, *Silent Poetry*, Princeton, New Jersey: Princeton University Press, 1995

Morgan-Jones, Ruth, *Hearing Differently: The Impact of Hearing Impairment on Family Life*, London: Whurr Publishing, 2001

Niemoeller, A.F., *Handbook of Hearing Aids*, New York: Harvest House, 1940

Orlans, Harold (ed.), *Adjustment to Adult Hearing Loss*, London: Taylor and Francis, 1985

Ree, Jonathan, *I See a Voice: Language, Deafness and the Senses – A Philosophical History*, London: HarperCollins, 1999

Sacks, Oliver, *The Man Who Mistook his Wife for a Hat*, London: Gerald Duckworth and Co., 1985

— *Seeing Voices: A Journey into the World of the Deaf*, Berkeley and Los Angeles: University of California Press, 1989

Soames, Mary, *Clementine Churchill*, London: Cassell, 1979

Spark, Muriel, *A Far Cry from Kensington*, London: Constable, 1988

Taylor, George and Anne Darby (eds), *Deaf Identities*, Coleford, Gloucestershire: Douglas McLean, 2003

Weston, Mark, *Working Without Hearing*, London: self-published, 2001

Wilson, E., *Shostakovich: A Life Remembered*, London: Faber and Faber, 1994

Wright, David, *Deafness*, London: Allen Lane, 1969

Wright, Tony, *Understanding Deafness and Tinnitus*, London: British Medical Association, 2003

SOME USEFUL NAMES AND ADDRESSES

UNITED KINGDOM

UK COUNCIL ON DEAFNESS
Westwood Park
London Road
Little Horkesley
Colchester
Essex CO6 4BS
Tel: 01206 274075
Fax: 01206 274077
Email: info@deafcouncil.org.uk

ASSOCIATION OF TEACHERS OF LIPREADING TO ADULTS
Westwood Park
London Road
Little Horkesley
Colchester
Essex CO6 4BS
Tel: 01206 274075
Fax: 01206 274077
Email: atla@lipreading.org.uk

BRITISH DEAF ASSOCIATION
1–3 Worship Street
London EC2A 2AB
Tel: 020 7588 3520
Fax: 020 7588 3527
Email: helpline@bda.org.uk

BRITISH SOCIETY OF HEARING THERAPISTS
Secretary: Dorothy Thomson
Hearing Services
12 Southend Avenue
Darlington
County Durham DL3 7HL
Tel: 01325 358185
Fax: 01325 469433
Email: dthearing@gofree.co.uk

BRITISH TINNITUS ASSOCIATION
White Building
Fitzalan Square
Sheffield
South Yorkshire S1 2AZ
Freephone: 0800 018 0527
Fax: 0114 258 2279
Email: info@tinnitus.org.uk

CITY LIT CENTRE FOR DEAF PEOPLE
16 Stukeley Street
London WC2B 5LJ
Tel: 020 7383 7624
Textphone: 020 7380 0416
Fax: 020 7380 1076
Email: CFDP@citylit.ac.uk

**DEFEATING DEAFNESS – THE HEARING
RESEARCH TRUST**
330–332 Gray's Inn Road
London WC1X 8EE
Tel: 020 7833 1733
Fax: 020 7278 0404
Email: info@defeatingdeafness.org

DISABILITY ALLIANCE
Advice, Research and Training
Universal House
Wentworth Street
London E1 7SA
Tel: 020 7247 8776
Fax: 020 7247 8765
Email: office.da@dial.pipex.com

DISABILITY RIGHTS COMMISSION
Freepost – MID 02164
Stratford-upon-Avon
Warwickshire CV37 9BR
Tel: 08457 622 633
Fax: 08457 778 878
Email: www.drc-gb.org

FOREST BOOKS
New Building
Ellwood Road
Milkwall
Coleford
Gloucestershire GL16 7LE
Tel: 01594 833 858
Fax: 01594 833 446
Email: www.forestbooks.com

HEARING AID COUNCIL
Witan Court
305 Upper Fourth Street
Milton Keynes
Buckinghamshire MK9 1EH
Tel: 01908 235700
Fax: 01908 233770
Email:
HAC@thehearingaidcouncil.org.uk

HEARING CONCERN
4th floor, 275–281 King Street
London W6 9LZ
Tel: 020 8233 2929
Fax: 020 8233 2934
Email: info@hearingconcern.org.uk

HEARING DOGS FOR DEAF PEOPLE
The Grange
Wycombe Road
Sounderton
Buckinghamshire HP27 9NS
Tel: 01844 348 100
Fax: 01844 348 101
Email: info@hearing-dogs.co.uk

**THE LINK CENTRE FOR DEAFENED
PEOPLE**
19 Hartfield Road
Eastbourne
East Sussex BN21 2AR
Tel: 01323 638 230
Fax: 01323 642 968
Email: linkcntr@dircon.co.uk

MUSEUMS AND GALLERIES IN THE CAPITAL (MAGIC)
c/o British Museum Education Dept
London WC1B 3DG
Fax: 020 7323 8855
Email: info@magicdeaf.org.uk

MENIERE'S SOCIETY
98 Maybury Road
Woking
Surrey GU21 5HX
Tel: 01483 740597
Textphone: 01483 771207
Fax: 01483 755441
Email: info@menieres.org.uk

NATIONAL ASSOCIATION OF DEAFENED PEOPLE
PO Box 50
Amersham
Buckinghamshire HP6 6XB
Tel: 01227 379538
Textphone: 01227 762879
Fax: 01227 379538
Email: enquiries@nadp.org.uk

ROYAL NATIONAL INSTITUTE FOR DEAF PEOPLE (RNID)
19–23 Featherstone Street
London EC1Y 8SL
Tel: 020 7296 8000
Fax: 020 7296 8021
Email: rnidmail@rnid.org.uk;
helpline@rnid.org.uk

SHAPE (ACCESS TO THE ARTS)
LVS Resource Centre
356 Holloway Road
London N7 6PA
Tel: 020 7619 6160
Fax: 020 7619 6162
Email: info@shapearts.org.uk

SIGNED PERFORMANCES IN THEATRE (SPIT)
1 Stobart Avenue
Manchester M25 0AJ
Tel/Fax: 0161 773 1715
Email: sarah@spit.org.uk

STAGETEXT
8th Floor
York House
Empire Way
Wembley
Middlesex HA9 0PA
Tel: 020 8903 5566
Fax: 020 8903 8647
Email: enquiries@stagetext.co.uk

BIRMINGHAM INSTITUTE FOR THE DEAF
Ladywood Road
Birmingham B16 8SZ
Tel: 0121 246 6100
Textphone: 0121 246 6101
Videophone: 0121 456 1535
Fax: 0121 456 6125
Email: enquiry@bid.org.uk

AUSTRALIA
AUSTRALIAN ASSOCIATION OF THE DEAF, INC.
Suite 513
149 Castlereagh Street
Sydney
NSW 2000
Australia
Tel: 02 9286 3944
Fax: 02 9286 3955
Email: aad@aad.org.au

**AUSTRALIAN FEDERATION OF DEAF
SOCIETIES**
101 Wellington Parade South
East Melbourne 3002
Australia
Tel: 03 6249 5144
Fax: 03 6249 8818
Email: tasdeaf@tassie.net.au

DEAFNESS FORUM OF AUSTRALIA
218 Northbourne Avenue
Braddon
ACT 2612
Australia
Tel: 02 6262 7808
Fax: 02 6262 7810
Email: deaforum@ozemail.com.au

NEW ZEALAND
DEAF ASSOCIATION OF NEW ZEALAND
PO Box 15770
New Lynn
Auckland
New Zealand
Tel: 09 828 3282
Fax: 09 828 3235
Email: national@deaf.co.nz

SOUTH AFRICA
DEAF FEDERATION OF SOUTH AFRICA
20 Napier Road
Richmond
Johannesburg
South Africa
Tel: 011 482 1610
Fax: 011 726 5873
Email: deafsa@icon.co.nz

UNITED STATES
NATIONAL ASSOCIATION OF THE DEAF
814 Thayler Avenue – Suite 250
Silver Spring
MD 20910-4500
USA
Tel: 301 587 1788
Fax: 301 587 1789
nadinfo@nad.org

GALLAUDET UNIVERSITY
Public Relations Office
800 Florida Avenue NE
Washington
DC 20002-3695
USA
Tel: 202 651 5505
Fax: 202 651 5698
Email: public.relations@gallaudet.edu

INDEX